Love, Luck And The Demon

John F. Roe

16pt

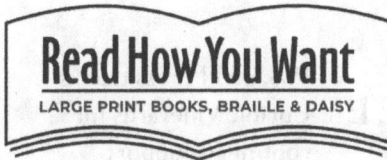

Copyright Page from the Original Book

Wakefield Press
16 Rose Street
Mile End
South Australia 5031
www.wakefieldpress.com.au

First published 2019

Cover designed by Liz Nicholson, designBITE
Typeset by Michael Deves, Wakefield Press

NATIONAL LIBRARY OF AUSTRALIA
A catalogue record for this
book is available from the
National Library of Australia

CORIOLE McLAREN VALE
Wakefield Press thanks
Coriole Vineyards for
continued support

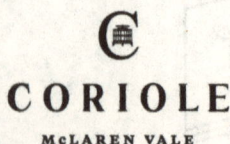

TABLE OF CONTENTS

Love, Luck and the Demon

Once Lincolnshire schoolboy, once Cambridge student, father, grandfather, teacher, writer, footballer, gardener, traveller – and once husband of Ella.

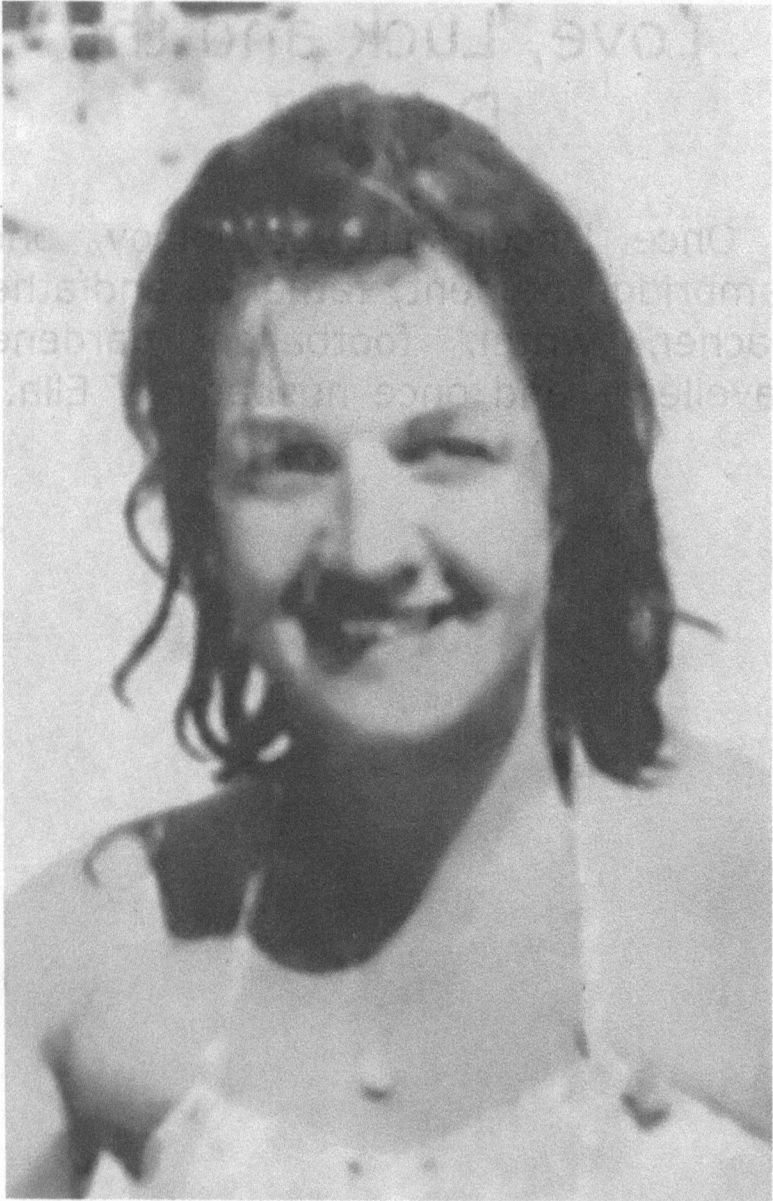

For
Alison Bennett and Madeleine Wilcock,
whose support made this book possible.

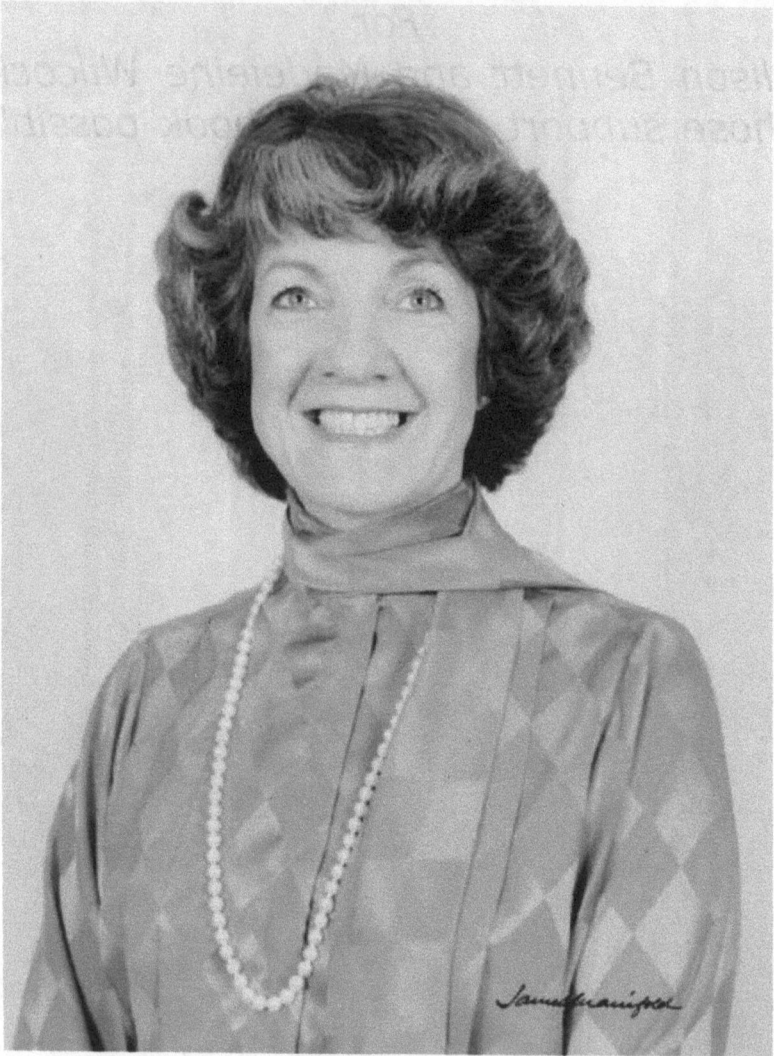

Ella Roe

I

This is a true story, all of it. Like all true stories it has no defined beginning or end and sadly maybe no significance, for there are really only two people in it and one is dead and the other often feels he died with her.

Where to begin? Let me tell you about the demon. The demon had a two-fold existence, appearing in the real world, often in disguise, and also in the shadowy world of nightmare. For some time, certainly more than a year, I never considered the possibility that the two demons were in fact one. The familiar one, the incubus, was enough. More than enough. We'll come to the daylight one later.

In outline and in action my nightmare was always the same. It certainly had no variety in its savage essentials, and at times it seemed almost absurdly to take satisfaction in reproducing tiny details: the same ornamental vase, the same chandelier, as in its numerous previous visitations.

Its central horror I understood well enough, but the dark world it inhabited still perplexes me for it lay within what was in essence unmistakably our home of forty-odd years in Skye, a hillside suburb of Adelaide. However, our house had expanded enormously. It was now three storeys high, not one, the ground floor being more or less the actual building, but overlaid upon it was a second storey somewhat resembling a long narrow ballroom, about fifty metres in length; it glittered with light and behind its arched windows seemed disproportionately opulent. It looked out over the city of Adelaide, and at times people, usually our friends, walked to and fro in this splendid room, often in lively conversation. Above this again was a third storey entirely of bedrooms, though our original bedrooms still existed on the ground floor. The garden, largely uncultivated, spread below the house on the natural slope of the hillside with no sign of the walls that now form terraces. The pool was still there, though not where it is in reality.

It was clearly a very large house, but it was exactly doubled in size by another building, also of three storeys, which adjoined our house and continued its line towards the east so that it extended into what are now other gardens in that direction. There seemed no neighbours anywhere nearby. This second building was tall, rectangular, largely of plate glass and apparently some sort of museum or antique shop, though on a grand scale with its three storeys all similar in size and proportions. Within it was a vast number of glass cabinets, each containing exhibits of objets d'art, generally ceramics, glass, porcelain, enamel and silver, often one to a shelf unlike the usual cheerful jumble of antique shops. It remained almost always completely empty of people, other than occasionally myself.

In the nightmare I leave the main house and reluctantly enter the exhibition, walking the length of its ground floor, up a spiral stair, then along its second floor, glancing occasionally at some eye-catching though coldly impersonal exhibit, before climbing another stair and so along the third floor to the very end. My progress, though never quick, grows slower as if the very air were impeding me. At the far end, now facing me, is a grey metal door. It exudes menace and hatred.

With a rush the demon emerges and my stomach churns and often I vomit. It seems to possess an electrical impulse for a fierce shock (exactly as a motor mower gave me as a boy) flings me backwards and the demon at once is on top of me. Its exterior is ill-defined as if cloaked in a greenish fog. As we wrestle I can sometimes feel, but with the external haze never quite distinguish, the physicality beneath. The demon's tactics are to lash me with gaunt clawed limbs, mine are to close through the green outer shell and land punches. My successes seem minimal compared to the wounds I take. On several occasions it claws out an eye (always the right eye) and usually tears deep gouges in my chest.

The confrontation begins again with the next nightmare. The struggle remains much the same. The details had only slight variations and I remember them well from between about 2010 and 2013. Though it is hard to recall the exact frequency of the clashes with the demon, they were rarely fewer than once per fortnight and sometimes more, even consecutive nights. The only variations came later, about the fourth year, when the demon seemed slightly less formidable, rather as if I had earned some token respect simply by showing up yet again for another harrowingly unequal grapple in the antiques establishment.

Recently, after many years and for no particular reason, I re-read John Bunyan's *The Pilgrim's Progress*. The story is, Bunyan tells us, 'Delivered under the similitude of a dream'. Christian, the central character, has a fearsome confrontation with the demon Apollyon. Walking in the Valley of Humiliation (and I've walked through that, I can tell you!) Christian 'espied a foul fiend coming to meet him ... Then did Christian begin to be afraid and he cast in his mind whether to go back or stand his ground.'

Of course, he stood his ground, going back being never an option. 'The monster was hideous to behold; he was clothed with scales like a fish ... and out of his belly came fire and smoke...' There follow threats from Apollyon, before the creature loses patience with Christian. Then Apollyon straddled quite over the whole breadth of the way and said 'prepare thyself to die ... here will I spill thy soul.'

It all sounded painfully déjà vu, particularly as then: 'Apollyon wounded him in the hand and foot', though not, I noticed, with masochistic vanity, clawing his eye out. 'Christian by reason of his wounds must grow weaker and weaker ... Apollyon wrestling with him gave him a dreadful fall.' In fact, Christian then fights back, stabs the monster with 'a deadly thrust' and it fled.

As a small boy I owned a child's copy of *The Pilgrim's Progress* with various wood-cut engravings. I always read it in bed. One engraving of Apollyon closing in on Christian was so macabre it made sleep difficult. That the monster straddled my future was not then mine to see. In no way did I consciously base 'my' demon (as I patronisingly called it) on Apollyon. If it lay for many decades in my subconscious it must have lain deep.

You have not heard the last of my dream (unless you cease to read here, which may have some merit) and two other dreams that appeared regularly, though less frequently than the one I have described, and during the same years. Both had as background the same huge three-storeyed house and the adjacent glassy cubes of the antique exhibition. Fortunately the demon was elsewhere.

In one of these lesser but very familiar dreams our large house, as in the demoniac nightmare, appears to be set about 1977 as the garden is unstructured, having no terraces and little if any cultivation, though the pool exists. In this dream it is invariably night-time (I never meet the demon by night) and I wake to hear, and soon to see, a bunch of thuggish vandals in the garden. They are mindlessly damaging things, uprooting the small shrubs and trees I've planted. Usually they try to wreck the pool, chipping the sides or smashing the filter. Clearly there are too many for me to confront them so

I try in the darkness to isolate a single thug and surprise him with fists and rocks. They always come in cars and park them on Knox Terrace, where it runs past the bottom of our drive. Sometimes, perhaps while they are mindlessly vandalising the pool, I damage their cars, usually thumping them with rocks. There appear to be five or six of them, with an evident leader whose face even now is vivid in my mind. I think it likely I've met him in my real life, but cannot recall how or where.

The third dream defies logic more than do the others, or at least my layman's logic. I find myself somewhere on Adelaide's North Terrace, but heading home on foot as urgently as possible. For some time, as I plod towards the hills, the scene is familiar, though the streets are unrealistically steep as they slope upwards. I can actually see our house, that is the dream-house, with its weird three storeys and the glossy façade of the antiques exhibition. Both are lit by bright sunlight but seem impossibly far and my determination to get there becomes pessimism: 'I'll never make it.' Then with one of dreaming's frustrating non sequiturs I find myself trudging along in some industrial factory town. Pressing in on me are looming factory walls, dark mills and endless claustrophobic workers' homes wherever I look. The going is harder now and the tall Orwellian greyness of it all has obscured our house completely. Indeed I have no sense of direction, yet do have a flash of understanding: this is Sheffield, in the north of England, a reasonable assumption based on my visits there in the 1950s, though today doubtless it has moved on from its *Road to Wigan Pier* days. Knowing where I am doesn't help my general dislocation, particularly as I now enter a random door and climb three sets of shadowy, musty stairs. Down a corridor a door opens and an elderly lady says, 'Come in then.' I go in. The room is frayed and faded. Everything is dusty and dimly lit. There is a younger lady, a daughter, I presume. Both ladies seem designed to repeat the room's attributes; the older lady wears a baggy beige dressing-gown.

The daughter says, 'You've come back.'

'I can't stay.'

'We've kept your room.'

'Thank you, but I need to get going.'

As always this and the previous dreams recreate themselves closely but not in perfect detail. For instance, in at least one variation of the third dream I recollect being offered a cup of tea. The demon itself never varies of course.

Dreamers among you may doubt the veracity of what you have read. The dreams did occur, occurred often, and with their frequency were easy to remember. That's all! They were what they were.

When my beloved wife died the dreams stopped. At once. Nor has any one of them re-occurred. As to when they began that is uncertain other than at some time in the last decade, so about 2010 or a little earlier. What I'm sure of is how frequently they afflicted me. It is tempting to say when asked of the wearying repetition, like some punch-drunk boxer asked to recall the blows he took, 'Oh, about a hundred, I suppose.'

In an old rural tale a farmer sets out to catch the moon in a net. Seeing the moon's perfect reflection in a pool of water he scoops it up. To his frustration it slips through the meshes and, as the water stills, the moon regains its watery shape. So my dreams slip through my memory, but I'll do my best to enumerate them: the dream of Sheffield, probably about fifteen times, the thugs in the garden, perhaps twenty appearances, but on a modest basis of twice a month for four years the phantasmagoria of the demon must have climbed towards a hundred.

May they never come back, though (why always these limitations?) once or twice I have found myself wishing I could really have it out with the demon, though again it's probably mutual. Maybe Don King could set it up.

II

I'm tired of talking about mental disturbance, for surely this must have been the engine that drove the dreams. So I'm going to tell you about a day I'll never forget, never! A real star of a day.

It was early in the July of 1954. My nineteenth birthday had passed in April and now was the beginning of the Long Vac, the four-month summer holiday from Cambridge. My exam results had just come; the exams had, as was not uncommon with freshmen, trapped me in a light-hearted and completely unjustified confidence. But I had scraped through and next year I meant to study hard. Cambridge was too good not to be there; all would be well. Now I was sitting in the Lincoln Tax Office on Silver Street starting a month's contract as a temporary file clerk. My next job through August and September was to be as a mill-hand in my uncles' mill. Having done this during the two previous summers the hard physical work was enjoyable as were the macho elements and the company of some tough workmates, one of whom had swum the Rhine to escape from Arnhem. But the harvest was not yet in so that job waited for a while.

The tax office would be boring and tame but it paid well. Day one started well too. The kindly Mrs Bosworth and Mrs Somers who ran the filing room gave me small easy jobs. The room was crammed with wall-shelves and cabinets and further standing shelves to the extent that the only place to sit down was on the window-sill. A single door opened onto 'our' desk on which various tax officers delivered completed files for us to store. As I sat on the sill the sun was warm through the window, the light as clear as my memory of the moment Miss Burley walked in.

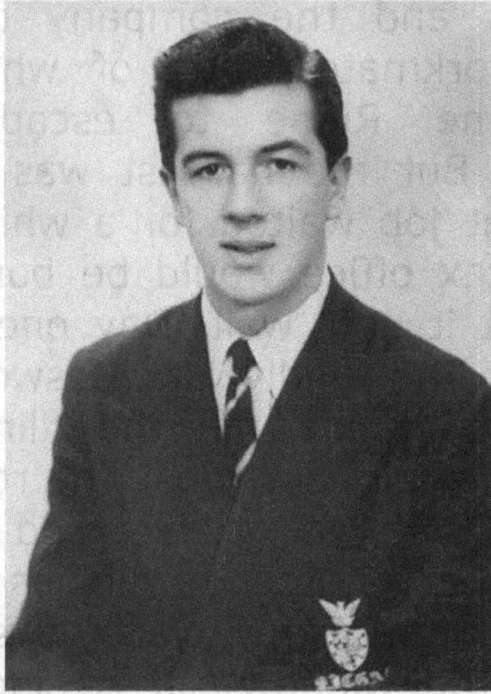

The young scholar: John Roe, October, 1953

'Are you our new filing clerk?' she said. 'Here are the Ruston files.'

Lincoln's major industry consisted of four great steel foundries and two of them were known as Ruston Bucyrus and Ruston and Hornsby. Together they employed a huge workforce and over the next hour or so Miss Burley and others brought in an enormous selection of the foundrymen's files. None of this meant much to me and inadvertently, but almost inevitably, I muddled the files of the two companies, my allocation going into a sort of generic Rustons collection.

Mrs Bosworth and Mrs Somers were disappointed in me. Miss Burley said, 'Oh for goodness sake!' with all the ring of Lady Catherine de Bourgh, though not adding, as did Lady C. in *Pride and Prejudice* 'I have not been used to submit to any person's whims. I have not been in the habit of brooking disappointment.'

Then the misplaced files began to flash into their correct niches with an effortless finesse, hers not mine, for which the word 'legerdemain' was surely created. 'Do you think you can manage now,' she said and left, her presumably rhetorical question echoing behind her. Miss Burley was wonderful. Everything about her. Everything! She was poised and dashing, her figure stylish, and she radiated a confident gloss, the sort of aura one sees in international athletes as they throw the victor's bouquet into the crowd. Add to this her hair was red, an eye-catching blood-red in a school-girlish pony tail, and her eyes were as blue as the summer sky.

'Are you all right?' said Mrs Bosworth. 'She can be a bit snappy.'

'I'm all right,' I said. 'She's OK.'

I would have broken the demon in half if it had laid a finger on her. I was a lot younger then.

The tax office was highly formal. The men were invariably addressed as Mr and only very junior girls appeared to have christian names. Even then etiquette called for these to be used only on certain occasions and then only by certain individuals. My naïve request to be told Miss Burley's first name was thus problematic. Mrs Somers released the information with a stricken look. It satisfied every criterion. She was called Ella. What else? Why the need to ask? The sweetest name in the whole cosmos, the proud name of the great Anglo-Saxon rulers.

The office's doctrines and cabals had no difficulty with my name. A low and temporary newcomer, propriety made me 'John' to the men though still Mr Roe to the ladies. At the time most of the people employed there seemed of late middle age. But two of the senior men were decorated fighter crew. In

1954 they could hardly have been more than in their late thirties, despite my impression that everyone was just short of retirement. The men and I had one strand of commonality: cricket. It was an unfailing fall-back for conversation and the office had its own team that played in a fairly serious evening competition. Could I play? A bit. Would I play? Of course, delighted.

The cricket was fun and several of the ladies came along as supporters. Miss Burley was away on a fortnight's training course and just as well. Run out twice wasn't likely to attract anything but a luke-warm pity. However fate's fickleness means that sometimes you just have to get lucky. Not often, I know, but that's the way it is. She was back from the course and came to watch the game. Fifty runs: oh bliss, oh thank you, destiny! Even a plumb LBW on three had been turned down.

At this point only one of us had spoken to the other, that being her obvious and one-sided disapproval of my incompetence at our first encounter. Despite the confidence-boosting runs there seemed no way to broach any sane conversation. It could hardly start: 'Did you see that innings of mine? My word, impressive wasn't it?' That gambit abandoned, no other sprang at once to mind. There was one gleam of light. Our skipper said that there was to be a team supper in a local restaurant. 'Hope you come along.' I had to. What if she went off on another course?

Looking back across the chasm that separates now from then I can hardly believe the sequence of events that were about to be provoked. I used to like playing roulette until my wife intervened (again more later). Sometimes I got on a run, always betting on red. When the ball whirred to a stop in a red niche it felt like a small victory. But now I wanted four reds in a row.

So I went to the supper not knowing whether Miss Burley would be there having found myself either too shy or simply too tongue-tied to ask. But she was there and the croupier paid out on the first red. Three to go.

I had brought along my cousin as company and support. This was a complex red but it might work. Tom was a year ahead of me at Cambridge, debonair and handsome. Please don't make a pass at Miss Burley. On the day he was unusually calm and made polite conversation. Another red.

I know the odds say fifty-fifty on every throw but it doesn't feel that way. My third red was to ask Tom to bring his father's white Jaguar. He had. Red again. I must have been mad.

Now for four in a row. That only happened to other people. Looking across the restaurant I saw Miss Burley among a coterie of girl-friends and Tom gave me a push. 'This is it, sahib,' he said and laughed. It didn't feel amusing. I moved forward stiffly, over the top now and into the gunfire of baffled expressions.

'Would you like to go for a walk, Ella?' I said. A second or two passed and I knew now how the defusing officers of World War II felt as they crouched over the ticking unexploded bombs.

She said something that I didn't quite catch, picked up her coat and walked around the table. Later she told me it was 'That will be nice'. I thought it sounded like 'Four reds'. Amazingly I have a photo (it's in the family album) snapped a fraction of a second before this moment by someone taking a general picture of the group. It is under my hand now. It feels archaic – maybe it's a daguerreotype – but it shows Guinevere having supper in Camelot among her ladies.

We extricated ourselves from a mix of wonder and suspended disbelief and walked out. Tom opened the door of the Jaguar.

'Whose car is that?' she said.

'My father's.' Tom helped me out.

'Well, you can take me home.' There was a pause. 'If we're going for a walk I want to change my shoes.'

We went to her house, a very short journey, and she changed her shoes probably, if later life was any guide, trying on forty or so alternatives.

Miss Burley's elder sister came out into the porch with her hair in curlers and gave the Jaguar a disdainful glance. At once I thought of the witch and the gingerbread house. I must be Hansel, and Ella Gretel. Tom wasn't so easy and didn't fit: just a lad with a white

Jaguar, conceivably out of *The Hitchhiker's Guide to the Galaxy.*

Tightening her curlers her sister said, 'You know she's engaged'.

'Don't be ridiculous,' said Tom dismissively, as one might on being told that bubonic plague had broken out next door. The sister went back inside, slamming the door, but her words hung in the porch.

Miss Burley emerged in changed shoes. I presume they were changed, they didn't look much different.

'Thank you for the lift,' she said, neatly disposing of her chauffeur who left revving the motor and shouting, 'John, you'll have to get the bus home.'

'Where shall we walk?' she asked.

'On the common, if you like.' This was a sweeping expansive grassland but no distance away, popular with sweethearts and lovers. We set off, slightly apart.

Encouraged by silence I said, 'Ella, are you engaged?'

'Don't be ridiculous,' she said.

Later I held her hand.

I don't know if you could call it a romance. I wouldn't. I'd call it a heartbreaking disaster with stupidity as its motif. We were to see each other only twice more, at least for years to come. There were to be two more walks and that would be it. One was around the grounds and battlements of Lincoln Castle where one of her school friends was the warden's daughter, thus free entry. Ella's money-managing skills approved of free entries. OK so far. The next walk replicated our first, that is on the South Common. At one point she stopped and took a photograph out of her bag. It was of herself, wearing a bikini and exuding glamour, on a beach shaded by palm trees. She produced a silver pencil and wrote on the back. I was pretty sure it was too early for 'Till death us do part' and indeed decorum was preserved with 'San Remo'. Her hands were small and warm in mine. This time she was audacious enough to kiss me. Once. I thought a butterfly had alighted on my lips.

The fourth rendezvous was to be at the main railway bridge in Lincoln. It's blurred now but I was about to take my life's most mortifying ill-starred action. The afternoon was sunny, my spirits were high, but she never came. I took the bus home and dialled her phone number.

'Where were you?' The facts were that the bridge was a triple span and very long and in a part of the city I hardly knew. I tried again, just about reaching 'Where...?' before the fury broke. She had waited (at the opposite end as it turned out) for an hour, yes, an hour, did you hear that, had never before been stood up on a date, didn't believe I had even been there at all, who did I think I was? It wasn't so much a tirade as a fuming, galling lecture on not being in the habit of brooking disappointment.

Any of an ounce of sympathy on my part or a shred of brain, even the word 'Sorry' might just have worked. Saying 'If you're going to take that attitude...' was the wrong response. By some margin.

The phone at the other end was slammed down for six years. Six and a half actually.

It is not absolutely accurate to describe my reaction to dismissal from Miss B's life as an anaemic surrender.

It is close to accurate, about ninety-nine per cent probably. But saying that would be to ignore the pheasant.

My shooting skills were good. From being quite young using an air-gun and then a .22 rifle seemed easy. Tom and I soon began shooting with his father's twin shotguns, out in the unkempt countryside that surrounded my uncle's remote farm. The shooting was enjoyable only in that it demanded skills and fast reflexes. The deaths I disliked and at nineteen, sickened by a maimed rabbit screaming, swore never to shoot another creature. Theoretically flies and mosquitoes should be exempt too but this mercy was better left to high-ranking Buddhists.

My very last shot was a fast reaction one, dropping a cock pheasant as it exploded unexpectedly from a small coppice. His turn now, my turn later. It was a beautiful bird, its plumage a dappled bronze with iridescent tail feathers.

'Let's go home,' I said to Tom. 'Drop in at Walnut Place for a minute or two.' Feeling almost half-witted I stood on her doorstep. The pheasant seemed incongruous, as if I might just as easily have substituted it for some other weird and colourful object, like a piano accordion.

Her mother opened the door, an unfamiliar lady but with her daughter's way of looking straight at you.

'I thought you might like this,' I said absurdly. 'I mean Ella might.'

'Thank you,' she said. 'It's a fine bird. She's not here. Would you like to come in and wait? She won't be long.'

'No, I've got to go.'

Thereafter nothing.

One would be entitled, indeed expected, to ask, given how fascinating I found Miss Burley, whether it was credible that it should be so airily terminated. In the words of Byron:

> 'tis strange the mind, that very fiery particle
> Should let itself be snuffed out by an article.

A phone call was, I suppose, a sort of article, but surely a bit more spirit and initiative was required, even a spell of walking meditatively past the Tax Office at lunch-time, 'alone and palely loitering'. But behaving in this forlorn Keatsian way somehow felt less than satisfactory, clearly having practical difficulties such as regular train journeys back from Cambridge to Lincoln, thus my studies hopelessly compromised and the consequent rustication. That word itself was enough: suspended from one's studies and sent off to a more suitable future as a country bumpkin.

To my surprise the sun continued rising and setting and nobody at all commiserated with me in my distress, though Tom did say 'Get a life'. Next there was my re-absorption into the consuming life at Cambridge (plus another rebuff from Ella). Then was the need to find a profession, these two demands lasting until about 1958, taking two years each. Then came the Betjeman girl, which consumed about three years. The fourth factor lasted about ten seconds and was a catastrophe of the nature of a giant asteroid striking the earth. At least.

Let me deal with them in the above order. Cambridge was both challenging and immensely enjoyable, particularly in the friends I made. At St John's

College my friends in a successful and talented soccer club decided in their usual casual fashion that in January 1955 they would reward their achievements with a footballing tour. There was a certain amount of debate on the basics, such as where to go and whom to play. Devon was no good, the cricketers had just been there, Durham was too far away, Wales was too dismal. Lincolnshire, I was told, would be perfect. This left to me the fixing of the matches and accommodation while the rest were able to enjoy themselves.

That January was bitterly cold and there were traces of snow on all the grounds we played at. But the matches were good and the accommodation and hospitality were marvellous, my parents having called upon the generosity of many of their friends. We were all based in Heighington, my home village, not far from Lincoln itself.

One night has stayed forever in my mind. It was mid-tour and the boys were congregating in their chosen pub, 'The Butcher and Beast'. Outside it was snowing gently, the flakes floating down at leisure, inside big fires blazed.

Someone (I'd never seen him before or since) sat at the piano and began to play. He was incredibly good and soon the boys began to sing. The songs were old but the voices were young.

I may be right, I may be wrong
But I'm perfectly willing to swear
That when you turned and smiled at me
A nightingale sang in Berkeley Square.

She had smiled – it didn't have to end here. Maybe...

There'll be blue birds over the white cliffs of Dover
Tomorrow just you wait and see...

Waiting and seeing hadn't done much so far.

Goodbye, Dolly, I must leave you
Though it breaks my heart to go...

Well, that said it all.

Frankie Gardner, the publican, flicked the lights off and on again, signifying time to close. The group's natural leaders were hard boys from Sunderland, Sheffield and Stockport.

They shook their heads: 'Private party isn't it, Frank?'

There's a long long trail
a-winding...
Until my dreams all come true

If only she'd just walk through the door. 'Another whisky, thanks.'

'Is she worth it?' said the boy from Stockport. He was reading Law – maybe there was a law against excessive sentimentality. The pianist seemed to know every tune on earth. Midnight came and went and our Welsh left-winger stood and sang solo:

After the ball is over, after the
break of morn,
After the dancers' leaving, after the
stars are gone,
Many a heart is aching if you could
read them all,
Many the hopes that have vanished
after the ball.

The girls behind the bar wept.

We'd fixed a dance, not quite a ball, in the Village Hall for the last night of the tour. I bought a gilt-edged invitation card and sent it to Walnut Place. She never came.

In later years I asked whether she ever got the card. 'Yes,' she said. 'I wish I'd come to the dance. I was too shy.'

There was a strange little postscript to the late night: in 2014 in England a man stopped me in the street and introduced himself. He had played against us on that tour and, can you believe it, had been in the pub that night, sixty years ago. 'Those Cambridge boys,' he said, 'they were crackerjack kids.' Two of them had only twelve years to live. Between them. Now the others have faded away. But they were crackerjack kids, all right. Shame my girl never met them.

She kept the invitation card. I know because it's in her little marquetry box in my study, with her other keepsakes.

III

Now for my profession: Cambridge behind me I felt unqualified for anything that came to mind. Like most people of my age I'd done plenty of casual work: a mill-hand (which I liked very much and was also the family business), postman, railway worker, grocery delivery boy, pea-harvester, potato-picker, even beet-singler, a job so laborious and mind-destroying that even thinking of it unnerves me. In all of these except perhaps the mill I'd reached an impasse which not only ruled out a future therein but somehow cast me as a dangerously unemployable eccentric. Delivering bread I had been attacked by a dog and had given it a well-merited kicking, leaving the Co-op grocery store unimpressed, as were British Rail when I high-mindedly helped an elderly and frail lady into her compartment, only to be carried away involuntarily from Lincoln to Doncaster (First Class). 'Oh young man, will you lose your job?'

'I hope so,' I said.

Somehow a Masters degree in history wasn't going to help in the avenues I had thus far explored.

The sane course would have been to take a Diploma of Education. Ella, finding herself in a somewhat similar situation, solved it by promptly going one better, taking a Degree in Education, but we'll come to that. The Diploma would take a year but would have given some rudimentary notion of teaching. Without any such qualification I foolhardily took the road less travelled. It led to Nottingham, or its western fringe, very close to the Erewash Valley, so unforgettably created by D.H. Lawrence in *The Rainbow.* There was a Lawrence museum that had been his childhood home within walking distance of my digs. My classes had not heard of Lawrence, being deeply concerned by the fortunes of Notts County FC (or more accurately 'Notts Count-eh', the latter a vowel sound hard to transcribe but addictive).

The school was a hard-bitten Secondary Modern. Towards the end of the year an inspector appeared charged with assessing my incompetence. His scrutiny suggested the verdict would be 'floundering'. My class were all fifteen years old; instead of their customary racket they were silent, stonily so, recognising a higher authority than mine. They understood hierarchy so now I was almost one of them. Disturbed by the absence of commotion though I was, the icing on the cake was hardly my fault. A crowned tooth popped out of my mouth (I think the word apostrophe caused it) bouncing high on a boy's desk immediately in front of me. Reflexively I caught and reinserted it. The inspector gazed, unsure of whether this dextrous move had really happened, and departed shaking his head. Only a couple of boys noticed.

'You should do that more often, sir,' one said.

The year I had lasted was longer than for several of my fellows. I nearly wrote 'fellow teachers' there but that would have overstated my case considerably. Time yet for a hundred indecisions, though beet-singling was not one of them.

My cousin Tom on leaving university had joined the RAF. He soon qualified as a fighter pilot, having all the appropriate panache, perhaps fostered by the white Jaguar. His aircraft was a Vampire. It stalled at one hundred feet up, his parachute had no chance of opening and the vampire sucked his life away. He didn't die. He was twenty-two then and is eighty-two now, but he'd give a lot for one day without pain. Just one. Or one day to walk. Just one.

Why mention this? Well, as I've related he played a small part in this story. I've not told you of my walking through black January nights, past Trinity College, past Kings, past the Fitzwilliam Museum down to Addenbrooke's Hospital where he lay in a cot shaking the rails, awake but unawake, knowing nothing.

I told him of many things that I've long forgotten, but I do recall (how inconsequential and how English) talking of 'off-breaks'. He would never bowl one again, nor any other delivery. A nurse came in and listened.

'Did he love cricket?' she asked.

'Yes.'

His broken body convulsed and the arm swung high, rattling the rails, almost as if swimming backstroke on the mattress.

'Keep talking,' said the nurse.

'He can't hear.'

'Yes, he can. Somewhere deep down. Keep talking about cricket.'

Fifty-eight years later another ward, another cot. For hours I spoke through tears to my heart's delight as she lay there.

'Keep talking. She can hear you,' the nurses said.

So I told her of love.

Putting all my savings in my pocket I shook off Nottinghamshire's coal-dust and hitchhiked in Europe for six months. It was partly enjoyable and partly tedious, notably when the three hundredth vehicle leaves you waving futilely outside Metz (yes, it happened). But so did being woken by cowbells tinkling in a meadow in the Pyrenees. Anyway down through Spain, over the straits, through the Atlas Mountains westwards. There were scrapes and scares but they didn't count for much, with one conspicuous exception. What did matter was the chance of a long air-borne hitch back to UK and then meeting Ann, the Betjeman girl.

Let me return to the conspicuous exception. This next segment was added considerably later when it became apparent to me that the 'exception' was part of the story after all, and not an irrelevance. Indeed it has the look of a non sequitur in the flow of events. It isn't, it's pretty central, so bear with me. The place was Algeciras. It hadn't much to recommend it, or so it seemed, except the view across the bay to Gibraltar. Getting a lift is a big deal for a hitchhiker, but it's not quite so good to arrive late at night. Better just to pull out your sleeping bag and find a sheltered spot in daylight under a tree or near a stream. Algeciras felt hot, cramped and full of mosquitoes. Was there anywhere to sleep? A down-at-heel hostel was offering beds, or mattresses actually, about six per room. It had to do. There was no light of any sort and sleep soon came. It was so hot the sleeping bag slid to my waist. Just as well.

At some point in the night I woke to feel hands around my throat. It is an eerie primitive feeling and for many men and women it's often their last. Try imitating it: just lightly put your hands around your own neck. My hands were free and I hit upwards instantly and savagely and felt the impact crunch into someone's face. The hands came away and feet ran to the door as I struggled free of the sleeping bag. No-one else woke, or at least no-one moved or spoke. The night passed in a doze, sitting upright with my back to the wall. The incident took a fraction of a second. I rarely think about it.

But something else happened, something really hard to describe. It was as if in a flicker, the last signs of adolescence had sped past. My response would have been fuelled by adrenalin, but it felt good. Perhaps the strangler would come back. So what? It didn't bother me. Nothing could hurt me now. It was as if my luck would never desert me. On a far greater scale my uncle when he got back from the killing fields of the Somme, having survived the battlefield's demons of guns and gas, may have felt something like that.

The demons (there are always two) of my story were still elsewhere. No doubt my little show of defiance in the dark room would be a triviality to them. Let's see if he can do it again, black night after black night, black year after black year. Demons win on black.

The Betjeman girl did what I thought damned difficult. She made me stop mooning over a predicament that had got all the action of a game of chess when both sides have black pieces. A consolation, small but you can't have everything, came from Dorothy Parker (she's a writer, not the Betjeman girl).

'And if he never came,' said she,
'Now what on earth is that to me?
I wouldn't have him back!' I hope
Her mother washed her mouth with
soap.

Actually I doubt whether either Sauron or He-who-must-not-be-named would have tackled washing Miss Burley's mouth out with soap.

Ann was small, delicate and pretty. Her expensive education at a girls' independent school had taught her nothing of an academic nature: 'I have only read one book in my life and that was *White Fang*. It was so frightfully good I have never read another'. Dorothy again, but could have been Ann.

But she was quick-witted and lively company. She was however, a single child, inextricably close to her parents, who lived affluently in affluent Surrey. If you read Betjeman's poetry, you and she will get better acquainted.

> *Fling wide the curtains, that's a*
> *Surrey sunset,*
> *Loud down the line sings the*
> *Addiscombe train,*
> *Leaded are the windows, lozenging*
> *the crimson,*
> *Drained dark the pines in*
> *resin-scented rain.*

Ann said I should meet her parents.

> *Her father's euonymus shines as*
> *we walk*
> *And swing past the summer-house*
> *buried in talk,*
> *And cool the verandah that*
> *welcomes us in*

To the six o'clock news and a lime juice and gin.

You will find that Ella and I several years later went off to Rhodesia. Ann would not have moved to adjacent unfamiliar Hampshire.

Penniless as I was, getting work was a financial necessity. Let's give teaching another chance. It was either that or busking and begging. A post came up in Essex. 'Where's that?' said Ann.

The post was for six months in Burnham-on-Crouch, with its salty feel, its boat-builder traders, its main street of weather-boarded cottages and Georgian houses. I should have got a job as an estate agent. But everything about it was great.

Well, nearly everything. One of my pupils, a sixteen-year-old gypsy girl who lived in a caravan camp farther down the river, developed a sort of crush and began standing outside Mrs Cohen's place, my kindly landlady. I can't recall the girl's name other than that it should have been, but wasn't, Dolores. Ella fitted Ella like a glove, so did Ann Ann, and the gypsy lass had all the torrid look of a Dolores.

'Please go home and do your homework.'

'Will you walk me back to the camp?'

'No, I've got to mark some exams.'

'Well, my Dad and my six brothers...'

Presumably they would be shortly making me an offer I couldn't refuse.

Let me say at this point that in no way whatever was my behaviour or sensual self-esteem akin to that, say, of Byron's Don Juan or for that matter Mozart's Don Giovanni. In parenthesis it was hard not to sympathise with the former; after all his spaniel and his tutor were both eaten by a hungry life-boat crew escaping a wreck. Thanks to his multiple affairs Don Juan was usually only just ahead of the game, and for me that was all too familiar.

Surrey was calling me back:

The Hillman is waiting, the light's in the hall,
The pictures of Egypt are bright on the wall.

My sweet I'm standing beside the
oak stair
And there on the landing's the light
on your hair.

My name was pointlessly on the waiting list for membership of both Sunningdale and Wentworth Golf Clubs. Who'd pay the fees? Ann bought me a boater for Christmas. Her parents hired the Trocadero for her twenty-first birthday. I had a very sore throat. An obnoxious doctor asked if I'd been inhaling 'substances'.

I said, 'Yes, fairy floss.'

'Is that a user's name for marijuana?'

'No, it's a user's name for Surrey.'

Finishing my contract in Essex I declined a tempting post in the Aleutian Islands, winning undeserved favour with Ann, and instead opting for a small unambitious grammar school in Sussex. Sussex was adjacent to Surrey and the names sounded not unalike. They were also alliterative and even a bit assonant. A bit. My options were narrowing down. Ann visited my parents who were captivated by her. Her Lincolnshire trip must have been arranged by World Wide Tours. To be honest the distance from Surrey was taken in her stride. She was never short of pluck. I liked her a lot.

Back in Lincoln for a couple of days I was punched violently in the stomach and fell to my knees gasping for air, knowing that as I got up another flurry of heavy punches would be landing.

Well, that's not true, but it certainly felt very like that. The beating happened outside the office of the *Lincolnshire Echo,* the local evening newspaper. Their office had a large window in which it displayed photographs of interesting items, such as a level crossing that was about to be demolished. Walking past I glanced casually at it, hoping for football photos. Her photograph was in the window: Miss Burley, Ella herself, looking serious but lovely and holding a large bouquet. Everyone else in the picture, about ten people, seemed very smartly dressed. There were other bouquets and a few children. Remember that the only other members of her family that I had thus far seen, and that only briefly, were her elder sister on the occasion of that lady's chilling malediction about engagement and her mother who had received the pheasant. I tried to work out the sequence and roles of the people in the photo, and indeed the consequences. Ella was dead centre, next to a smallish man, formally dressed, then on either side other girls in white, some little ones at the front and book-ending the picture two pairs each of a formal lady and gentleman. The truth was plain to see, of course. She was the bride. I walked away distraught, though why this should be the case considering our minimal and clearly terminated involvement is not easy to see.

I had always sympathised with the Wedding Guest whom the Ancient Mariner had semi-hypnotised into listening to his dirge of a tale. Now even more was this the case as it came back to me how:

> *He* [the Wedding Guest] *went like one that hath been stunned and is of sense forlorn,*
> *A sadder and a wiser man he rose the morrow morn.*

Well, maybe not wiser but you can't have everything. Nor would I have gone to the wedding in the unlikely event of having been invited.

Surely life would be sadder. And it was. Ann clearly knew nothing of the cataclysm and certainly had she known couldn't have cared less. She had never been told a word of Miss Burley, but guessed instinctively that I'd had my fill of Lincoln. I was told I needed a holiday, had clearly been working too hard. We went to Monte Carlo together, her mother seething with disapproval. The casino was pretty ritzy and functional enough to relieve me of twenty pounds (exactly a week's wages). In a moment of insight I'd placed it all on black. Red was for someone else.

Surrey had just won the county cricket championship. They always did. It must be a pretty good place. Equitation might be the way to go. Showjumping or cross-country events would be asking too much, but anyone could do dressage, surely. Ann said, 'Don't be silly' and taking pity added, in her cut-glass accent, 'Look, no-one's asking you to change your name to Jolyon.' Both the future and certainly the immediate past looked to be slanting downhill, despite Ann's brio.

A telling off, three walks, one kiss and one caustic phone call. My elder grandson would say, 'Get over it', and the younger one declare: 'It is what it is.' But only a time machine could reach them.

So obviously she was now gone forever. I had to get over it, so gathering every penny and a hefty overdraft I bought a new car. Driving didn't interest me much, not as it does for many young men, nor was it a rite of passage. My earliest experience of driving was actually on a tractor and regularly I used to double declutch in cars. I'd driven bread vans, lorries and even at Cambridge an antique London taxi, co-owned with my cousin Tom, and had survived a crash that wrote off my father's car. All this was before acquiring a licence. Licences and tax returns were frustrations and could be dealt with in some indeterminate future. My previous car caused other motorists to wind down windows, point, and break into laughter. It was registered to a travelling zoo and was abandoned one night in a railway station car park. It may still be there.

As I said, I bought a car. It was an Austin Healey sports car, shiny and powerful and my lucky red. Ann was delighted with my purchase and bought me some racing-driver gloves. She would frequently drive it herself, the hood wound back, always with reflecting sunglasses and a silk headscarf. We went to a regatta and a flower show. My star was on the rise, at least in Surrey.

Her parents were perplexed by my new acquisition (i.e. the car not the gloves). To them I was and remained a social anomaly. My father was a substantial land-owner, my mother a nationally known pianist. I was on Christian name terms with two earls, several viscounts (Cambridge was full of them) and a cricketing Indian prince, inevitably known as Ranji. Why then was I employed as a small-town chalkie with leather patches on the elbows of my sports jacket? My future could at best be a doddering Mr Chips. What meant also my practice of playing football for aggressive downtown teams in the anonymous fringes of North London? Pre-eminently, why smoke Woodbines or even the unspeakable Gauloises? Ann and her mother both smoked Peter Stuyvesant, cork-tipped. Did I intend, with their daughter, to join a commune?

Their confused image was not unlike my own, my life having neither focus nor rudder. What prospect was there of steering it towards Miss Burley, now an unreachable Mrs X? That our fleeting acquaintance had clearly meant little to her was understandable enough, that it had meant so much to me defied all logic. Get a grip. It is what it is.

IV

As so often consolation came from elsewhere: from Shoreham Boys Grammar, West Sussex, or at least the boys thereof. They were my fourth group of pupils and, unsurprisingly, the three previous groups had taught me substantially more than I them. Doubtless vast numbers of young men and women, as gauche as I was, would have said the same after their first fumbling attempts to enter adulthood or, indeed, the teaching profession.

All our most holy illusions were
knocked higher than Gilderoy's kite,
We have had a jolly good lesson
and it serves us jolly well right.

Kipling's lesson was one that the Boers around 1900 had taught the antiquated British Army of the day. Mine was much the same. Trying to mimic those who taught me as a boy was not without merit, but long term wasn't going anywhere. In fact I'd been astonishingly lucky with my teachers. Four of them, Mrs Williams and Miss

Cox at Heighington Primary, and at sixth form level Mr John Hudson and Mr Alec Wood were inspirational. About ten people in my life worthy of that word have crossed my path – and four taught me! Four balls in the red slot when the stakes were high. You'd take that wouldn't you?

I doubt that the Betjeman girl had been that lucky. Miss Burley, I discovered later, had scored about the same as I had.

It was clear enough that my novitiate in Nottingham had been a failure. It deserves and will receive no further comment. The two spells in Essex were different. The differences were utterly different – if you see what I mean. The Essex schools were co-educational. This forced me to recognise the existence of two sexes, or rather that on one side were my mother, my grandmothers, sister, Ann and Ella, while on the other several billion boys and men. It seemed desirable to have two modes of teaching, one for the stoicism of the boys, another for the girls who seemingly had a far more extended spectrum of emotion. There were tears: 'It's my party and I'll cry if I want to' and there was recrimination, unlike the boys who circled the wagons in the stubborn voortrekker way. The girls also had a way of looking as if they all shared some secret which lay well in their futures and alongside which pedagogics was at best an amusing trifle. The gypsy girl, remember her, did this to perfection. Thankfully her caravan moved on and with it the remote possibility of an alliance based on her divining tea-leaves and me making clothes pegs. 'Men are from Mars, women are from Venus' seemed at the time a self-evident axiom. It is, of course, nonsense. The excoriation Miss B had dished out over the phone had red planet written all over it.

The very first novel I recall reading was *Ivanhoe,* a fact that still amazes me. No earlier involvement with fiction returns to mind unless one counts *Peter Pan and Wendy.* Rebecca, supposedly the lesser of the two heroines of *Ivanhoe,* was a real handful often seeming to disrupt the novel's plot. The Essex girls had a lot of her unsettling disposition. So when the post in Sussex became available its being all boys would surely make things easier, if only on the simple pretext that one gender would be easier to instruct than two. Whether this was or ever is the case remains uncertain, to me at least, as always thereafter my classes remained only boys. It didn't concern me a lot, anyway.

However something else happened. As usual with youngish newcomers (I was twenty-four) they aren't given much choice of their hierarchical rung. My classes were all juniors and academic battlers. They supported, in a relaxed way, Brighton and Hove Albion FC and were easier company than the hardline supporters of Notts County. So, unhassled by discipline problems and not now confused by the oblique perspectives of the girls, the lessons began to make sense. What was strange was that the successful lessons were on the English language and its literature, rather than on History. Furthermore in those two years in Sussex my reading became voracious and close to obsessive. My knowledge of English literature was minimal, without exaggeration. My school had virtually ignored any form of it. In those two years my mind became saturated with Dickens, Hardy, George Eliot and Jane Austen, starting in the nineteenth century only because I had to start somewhere; then came Wordsworth, Coleridge, Byron, Shelley and Keats, who were not only fine poets but all seemed to know one another and behaved like characters in a play. The school's boarding-house provided an apartment and meals, so plentiful leisure time favoured this new passion. I read *Macbeth,* never having read it before nor seen it on stage. It was intoxicating. I rushed out and bought it on an LP.

This is not a biography. It is not. If anything it is the story of the demon which at this time did not concern me, never having explicitly heard of it, though I had heard of Auschwitz, which sounded the sort of name a demon could have, better probably than Apollyon. In any case the demon was elsewhere busy tormenting ordinary decent people to meaningless despair and eventually death. Its story is this story. Honestly.

As 1959 and 1960 passed I naturally visited my parents and siblings in Lincolnshire. This brought me close to Ella geographically and from time to time I must have thought of her and wished her well. She was only a memory and would stay that way. Life wasn't always roses.

Then quite suddenly she re-appeared, on three separate occasions, into my life. The first of these lasted perhaps a couple of minutes, the second was a sort of contact in absentia, the third and most disturbing took something like five minutes. What occurred had all the feel of chance at work, as was usual in my life, rationalise it how I would.

My father became a director of a large grain company. Among his responsibilities were the general cash flow and, wait for it, tax. Casually he told me he was taking the employees' tax details to the head office. Would I give him a lift? Yes. 'That young Miss Burley soon sorts them out.' What was happening? It transpired that my father and his company had previously dealt with Miss Burley 'who knew what she was doing.' This statement needed more time to analyse than I had available. 'Yes Dad, I'll bring the files in for you.' Yesterday leave me alone.

We entered the office and she appeared. There was no catching her eye, my father having all her attention. After several minutes, he, she and the files said farewell. My own muted goodbye presumably merited, and certainly got, no more than an uninvolved glance.

The second occasion was equally unproductive though rather different. By this time I had worked both casually and in the teaching profession, though often for shortish spells, for roughly six years and had never filled in a tax form. Indeed since the heyday of July 1954 I don't recall having seen one. They occupied that fraction of my attention that differential calculus or basket-weaving does now. 'I've given what I could find of your financial details to Miss Burley,' said Dad, tired of requests in buff envelopes, since I always gave officialdom my home address, unless I was there. Some days later he handed me a cheque. 'She knows what she's doing, that young lady,' he said in an admiring, rather repetitive way.

'Isn't she married now?' I ventured.

'Bound to be, I suppose. She's never told me. I've always called her Miss Burley.'

At least she would be unconcerned by my tax labyrinth, other than that it confirmed my general fecklessness. Anyway that was what she told me in the unpredictable future that awaited us both!

Then things took another step, though in which direction was debatable. Football fixtures brought my local team, with whom I still played occasionally, into Lincoln. Sometimes it seems, I have measured out my life with football fixtures.

The younger members of this team had, earlier that year, distinguished themselves by organising a sort of fair, which, far from raising money, almost sent the club bankrupt. Five decades later those involved still remembered it as the fête worse than death. The lads involved believed they were sophisticates and irresistible to ladies and persuaded me to drink gin and synthetic lime at the supposedly upmarket Saracen's Arms before going with them to the supposedly genteel Co-op Ballroom. She was there. The flame of her red hair dimmed everything else. She was dancing like a Valkyrie, fast and furious, the rock and roll beat that she loved, not that I knew it then. When the music stopped she retired sedately to a line of chairs, cooling her face with her handkerchief used as a fan. Young men gathered near her though none had the narrow face in the wedding photograph. The band struck up some Latin American tune; she was on her feet transforming the Co-op Ballroom into Cordoba.

Under threat from Ann I had recently attended dance classes but knew my limitations well. The simpler patterns of waltz and quick-step were manageable, but the maze of manoeuvres for anything else was too daunting. 'Take your partners for the last waltz', said the band-leader. As she walked nearby I stepped across her path. 'May I have this dance, please?' I must have said that or something like it: you see it is close to fifty-seven years ago now. She took easy steps, rather as I would one day throw easy balls to tiny boys with bats. We circumnavigated the ballroom once before speaking.

'I saw you come in,' she said. 'I never thought you'd ask me to dance.' She still kept the steps simple, in perfect time.

'Thanks for doing my tax returns.'

'They were a shambles,' she said, rather limiting that unimaginative line of talk. She was wearing a silver-grey dress with tiny black specks. It was one of her favourites and she wore it often in the years to come. It fitted tight and, with her sleek figure inside the silvery sheath, felt as fluid as if in my arms were a seal or a mermaid.

'Are you alone?' Silence: so try again. 'Could I give you a lift home?' For a moment the ball hesitated over the red slot.

'Thank you, but no.'

I'd probably got off lightly. Being beaten up by the local bravos for seducing a neighbourhood girl had no appeal. The Austin Healey would be a red rag to the district's sans-culottes. Before the rough stuff started they would almost certainly ask me who I thought I was and would not take kindly to my preferred response of 'The Duke of Devonshire'.

'I'm afraid my father's waiting. He's walking me home.' The band were packing their instruments as I watched her leave. It didn't make sense. Alone? No particular partner? With her father?

The true and unpalatable state of affairs was beyond me, there to remain until March 1962, a year hence.

V

As boys and girls in Lincolnshire, and one knew few other places in those untravelled days, our thoughts and hopes were, as with all our contemporaries, formed around 'home'. So for Ella, 'home' was Walnut Place. How could it be otherwise?

Let me quote from Simon Schama's *History of Britain*. It helps.

British terraced houses were based on the nuclear family unit, perhaps with extended families such as uncles, aunts and grannies, as well as neighbours, congregating in back gardens and sometimes on the street, and in local shops, churches and pubs. Rooms were separated by function – kitchen, living rooms, bedrooms, and in the better or more socially ambitious houses, a parlour seldom used except for special occasions and to display domestic treasures such as the piano and sideboard. Like gas for lighting and cooking, water was now supplied municipally and delivered through taps directly into sinks instead of through an outdoor pump. Water closets were fast replacing earth closets...'

Schama got it close, except there was no garden at 6 Walnut Place, nor at any other house in that and a host of terraces of which it was part. The front of Number 6 was a rarely-used façade facing a narrow road. Everyone lived at the back. The terrace went back to back with Lime Grove, separated only by a narrow path which ran between the minute walled yards of each row. The folk of the area were frequently three-generational and Ella's grandma lived next door. The boys married the girls they played with, rarely venturing outside the gene pool. Each knew what his or her partner would bring. There was a wealth of traditional skills, some of them among the seamstresses dating back centuries. There was insularity and wariness of unlike societies, of those that lived differently. The young ones, at eleven years old, spotting an exit they weren't sure they wanted, poured disproportionately after 1944 into the new academies in the city. The boys were often small and wiry, older than their years, the girls quick to bloom, quick to age.

There was pride: we're downtown, we can lick anyone from anywhere, with fists or footballs, and that's just our girls. And they're our girls, get it? I spent eight years in school with these boys. It's how they thought, believe me. But there was affection, perhaps not romanticised and the clinging self-reliant loyalty of the bees in the hive.

Number 6 Walnut Place had the unvarying two bedrooms, in one of which the three sisters slept. The pressure to move out, particularly to marry, must have weighed heavily. There were two rooms downstairs, though the 'parlour', so called, was for some time occupied by a mysterious elderly and frail man, the landlord, I suppose. So the family chiefly used one downstairs room and in it lived, cooked, bathed in a tin washtub, played, Ella and Janet did their homework plus a thousand other things. There was gas, running water, but no fridge. Outside was a toilet, unlit and icy in the cold nights. Always on Mondays a fire was lit under a boiler, and the water was used for laundering, while in the evening more water was heated for the family to bathe in the tin tub. Mrs Burley cooked skilfully in a tiny space and when enough of her children had left home even took in a lodger. As the children entered the workforce they paid rent.

Here is where we go backwards. In general it's a better place to be, not always admittedly, but listen to this:

Into my heart an air that kills
From yon far country blows:
What are those blue remembered hills,
What spires, what farms are those?
That is the land of lost content
I see it shining plain,
The happy highways where I went
And cannot come again.

Those blue hills and church spires have a certain bucolic appeal but they don't matter much except as a sort of generic metaphor. One could substitute 'grey remembered terraces' for the hills and 'factory chimneys' for the spires and it loses no relevance. 'Happy highways' doesn't need any modification at all.

Little Ella ran, played, laughed and cried in the tight grid of small streets that intersected the foundrymen's houses. Like a geometric spider Walnut Place lay at the heart of the maze. The streets were so self-duplicating that the only way an outsider like me could penetrate the web was by searching for street names, names on plaques so grey as often to be indecipherable. Even years later I would get lost, particularly when one-way streets were imposed.

Only briefly had the family left the area, her mother inexplicably taking them all down to London to lodge with an aunt in a house adjacent to Crystal Palace's football stadium, only to be driven back northwards by the bombing for this was 1942. Back in Walnut Place was safety and outside the door was the familiar tarmac, paving stones, cobbles and 'kick-the-lamp relievo'. This game, for I took it to be a game, was and remains a mystery. As such it ranks right up with the Giant Rat of Sumatra, one of Holmes's most testing cases, about which Dr Watson chose not to elaborate. Ella did elaborate much later on the business of the lamp and it still meant nothing to me other than that it involved torches and screaming, always in the dark, before mothers fetched in their female offspring. Boys were verboten.

By daylight there was roller-skating, make-shift go-carts to race and learning to ride on ancient adult-sized bicycles. There was also skipping, more an art than a game, having degrees of proficiency, and in the street she skipped, her feet a blur, on and on into the twilight.

Her elder siblings moved out and now it was she who shopped and learned that two pennies bought only few sweets so shop carefully. All this time the war raged on and she with her mother stood in the alley outside their home and screamed encouragement upwards as the great black Lancasters roared across the skies of Lincoln, navigating on the cathedral's towers. Lincolnshire was the pre-eminent bomber county and Bomber Command was always special for her. As the Lancasters returned towards dawn, sometimes limping back, often tattered and with engines spluttering, even with one or two silent, mother and daughter, side by side, shrieked, 'Go on, go on, you can make it!'

In her happy years she told me of all these things and I told her of the night my mother woke me and led me into the garden to point out a red glow spread on the horizon. 'That, John,' she said, 'is the city of Hull and it's burning. Take my hand and swear that one day you will burn their cities.' Nervous of her intensity I promised. As things turned out I was spared the demons of flak across the dark night and the unthinkable horror of the flaming crash. Hugh Dickinson was in my primary class. His brother Aubrey burnt in the fire over the city of Nuremberg.

My father was about this time with the Eighth Army in Italy. Ella's father was then RSM of the Gold Coast Regiment in Africa. My father was generous and big-hearted. 'The Germans were fine soldiers,' he said one day at the dinner table years later. My mother, whose brother had drunk the gas on the Western Front, walked out of the room with a hiss like a snake, leaving us eating in an anxious silence, an early childhood lesson that 'the female of the species is more deadly than the male'.

Twice Ella hissed with fury at someone while with me. Both targets were women and each knew the rage at once for what it was. Men she tended to ignore in similar situations on the sure and certain grounds that they knew no better and that it was therefore up to me to rebuke them.

The RAF touched my own life in an odd little way in 1942, when my parents sent me to live for a while with my lonely grandmother. She had an RAF ground-crew man billeted on her. One of his tasks was to help camouflage Waddington, a huge bomber aerodrome close enough to my home for me to see its lights from my bedroom window. Francis and I lit bonfires far enough away from the aerodrome to divert the Luftwaffe, or so we hoped. They were eerie nights, driving down forgotten lanes, across untended fields and through sweeps of bracken to set alight log-piles. Francis would enliven the night by reciting poetry, usually of a patriotic-imperial genre such as *Gunga Din* or *The Relief of Lucknow* or *The Green Eye of the Little Yellow God*.

Little Ella, and she was always the smallest of her covey of girlfriends, did far more onerous work, jobs that today sound too laborious for an eight- or nine-year-old. One was fetching coal. Coal came from the coal-yard where trains dumped thousands of tons of it. That meant going there to collect it. It came loose or in sacks. A sack could be wheeled home across a bicycle's handle-bars or dragged on a home-made cart. On a couple of occasions the area flooded and she took the big tin bath, floated it to the coalyard, filled it as much as possible without it sinking and hauled it back home.

Lying in bed together luxuriating in its warmth, for that was invariably where she released her history, she would say, 'I bet you had it easy'. Up to a point that was not inaccurate but to dispel her notion of my adolescence of sybaritic ease it was necessary to relate the weight of the grain-sacks I carried across my shoulders in the

Heighington mills, aged sixteen: eighteen stone wheat, sixteen stone barley. 'Men are OK at that sort of thing,' she would concede. The taxing problem of navigating coal through floods clearly required something more enterprising than merely lifting bags.

Her longest job, that went on for several years from about eleven to sixteen, was delivering newspapers. The *Lincolnshire Echo* was a widely-read local evening paper. Our girl delivered a hundred copies on every night except Sunday and on Saturdays did a second shift of eighty or so *Football Echo*'s. Every copy was pushed into a letterbox. To do this required a total familiarity with Walnut Place and its surrounds. Many of the deliveries were in narrow alleys and often into dark tunnels where even she admitted to feeling nervous. Daylight, darkness, wind, rain and snow the papers had to go out and that for five years. When asked whether she regretted the time spent in this years-long chore she laughed. 'I bought a gold watch with the money,' she said, 'and at Christmas there were tips and as many mince pies as I could carry home.' I have the watch now – it is tiny and exquisite: looking at it makes me shiver.

Then there was school, St Andrew's Primary to be exact. From the little revealed to me it seemed like rather a good school in an austere sort of way. The arts were difficult to find and music less so, which tallied exactly with my own experience. What were taught and very thoroughly were the three 'R's, the children chanting seven-eights-are-fifty-six or developing a copperplate style of writing.

However there were other sources of learning for the children of that time and place: Sunday Schools and the Church itself. Both left their mark. She sang as a chorister in St Mark's Anglican Church until she was twenty-seven and must have met a thought-provoking Christianity as the parish priest was Oswald Jones. Oswald was my school's chaplain and a famous charismatic, not to say galvanic, preacher.

Another co-incidence (they are mounting up and I am not sure they are as random as they appear) was that my mother was for years the organist at St Mark's. When asked later whether she knew the all-important redhead in the choir she remarked disappointingly that organists concentrate on playing.

VI

Feeling restricted at Shoreham I applied for a post in Cleethorpes, an odd town in that it conjoined another town, Grimsby, with no apparent boundary, yet neither township appeared remotely aware the other existed. Cleethorpes looked to provide holidays for the northern industrial workers and in that role was decidedly unambitious. The beach was not unpleasant but the sea was grey and cold. The beachfront played host to a long line of tawdry stalls offering the opportunity, for a few pence, to make machines disgorge small combs or packets of gum. It was called Wonderland. Grimsby was appropriately grim, but had its highly-regarded trawling fleet. The remainder of Lincolnshire, solidly farming country, lumped both towns together as a sort of beach-head from which invading aliens had yet to break out.

In this gritty enclave I was to find, for the first time, the exhilaration of teaching, which few people understand. For a youngish schoolmaster there was still the uncertainty of knowing that one's audience might lose, or never even gain, faith in their appointed instructor. Sometimes one sensed, as the tight-rope artist knows half-way across Niagara, that there must be easier ways to earn a living. The school itself was very different from my earlier ones, in fact closely resembling my senior school in Lincoln, being academic but unadventurous, though with an unpredictable headmaster. My classes, all being the product of a selective system known as the eleven-plus, were bright enough. The school recklessly gave me two top examination classes. One was the Oxbridge scholarship class which was daunting as they had opted for Shakespeare's history plays as their special topic. Despite my fervent, haphazard reading this area had mostly escaped me, though I had in my boyhood seen the film *Henry V*. They were smart boys – they must have been as they sailed through.

But 5A, my favourites, lay elsewhere. They inhabited a dark utilitarian room. It had the usual pre-war desks work-scarred and inked, the walls bare and spartan. Our lessons were often in the late afternoon when, outside, dusk closed in and often brought fog. Inside we engaged in a thirty-person process of groups or even individuals pushing to usurp one another's territories. The alliances and commitments changed unpredictably. Two of the competing groups remain in my memory: one, a supposedly anarchic clique of Mick Wadsley, Steve Woodhead and their mates needed to be both entertained and contained, and another was the boys from the fenlands, who purported to be primevals not trifling with academia. There is no leisure in a crucible or they and I might have spoken of beet-singling.

My teaching technique (if one may be so lofty) as usual was much akin to Lucky Jim's scrambling to stay ahead of the game. Lacking an orderly core knowledge of literature and short of formal certainty with language (what was the subjunctive anyway?) my approach became a sort of pyrotechnics that may, for some at least, have brought their set texts to life. Anyway, I hope so. The Merchant of Venice was our Shakespeare: would the Third Reich have railed Shylock into Dachau? Was usury a sin? It was deemed so in Elizabethan England, yet the Globe Theatre was built on a ten per cent loan. Venice was neither a pantomime place nor a tourist stop, it was a grand empire; their fleet had hammered the seemingly unstoppable Ottoman Turks at Lepanto in 1571. Who lost one arm in the fighting? Anyone know? Cervantes. Who wrote what? Yes, Merrick? Sir, Don Quixote. Well done, published 1605, seven years after *The Merchant of Venice,* same year as *Macbeth.*

Antonio and Bassanio must often have walked past the world's greatest shipyard at the time, the Venice Arsenal. Arsenal? The heads came up: 'Was Arsenal FC called after...?'

'Of course, McCracken.' You can see that both my grasp and method were rather like lightning limning the clouds' dark edges.

Did my classes, particularly my crucible class, sense this gowned dilettante in front of them was amusingly illuminating but a little short of substance? The class's alignments changed unpredictably; for instance the fenlanders became my allies on hearing of my sympathy for The Pilgrimage of Grace when their ancestors, also people of the fens, who weren't short of a gritty obstinacy, paid a dreadful price when they objected to having their religion aborted to pay Henry VIII's debts. Allies were helpful when metaphorically I was struggling to hold together a ramshackle confederacy.

Remember where we are in time: until my thirty-third year I'd rarely seen a television, let alone any of the multiple devices that have joined it in claiming our attention. Films were not unfamiliar, but above all the medium was print. Buy books in paperback, read them, loan or give them to my pupils, let boys and books loose on one another, a constant whirlpool of reference, inquisition and diversion. Among a festoon of titles came *1984, The Heart of Darkness, Fahrenheit 451, Catch-22* (published that very year 1961, the same year Hemingway shot himself), *The Old Man and the Sea, The*

Great Gatsby and the weird poignant *Gormenghast,* just to name a few.

In fact the class felt its own zeitgeist was best expressed in a film: *A Rebel Without a Cause.* There was resistance to my claim that this was nothing new:

> *An if we live, we live to tread on kings,*
> *If die, brave death, when princes die with us.*

'That's Hotspur, lads, the real deal in the rebel spectrum.'

'Sir, are Tottenham Hotspur...?'

'Bound to be, Wilkinson.'

Had I known it, James Dean, the rebel himself, was much admired by Ella. Disappointingly she denied that Dean and I had anything in common. 'You've got a cause,' she said. She was right, though she misconstrued it.

The second half of 1961 passed and then in March of '62 everything changed. And what's more for the better. As far as my amours were concerned it was high time. The long-delayed moment arrived quietly and accidentally. The earth didn't move under my feet or not far, not yet. There was no sense of volcanic upheaval. Perhaps this was just as well as Ann had finally settled our embattled relationship, delivering a simultaneous *coup de grace* and *coup de théatre* with an air of long-tried patience ending: 'You have some good qualities, I'm certain, but when Mother said you might be getting a tattoo it broke my heart.'

It was a Saturday morning and chance and my own mother had sent me shopping in Lincoln, casually carrying an empty basket. It was on Silver Street close to the acclaimed Tax Office and she came walking along the pavement towards me. It had the same effect on me that our previous fleeting encounters had, that is preventing whatever one said from having any resemblance to one's thoughts.

I did manage to find enough savoir faire to say 'Hello' and Mrs X, as I tried not to think of her, replied 'Hello.' It was eerily like my French oral exam at school, when I greeted my lady examiner with '*Bonjour*' to which she replied '*Bonjour*'. Unable to conjure anything remotely conversational I said gravely, '*Bonjour encore*', at which the lady smiled and said, '*Quelle politesse!*' Thereafter things, I'm glad to say, improved.

So it did that morning. Together we walked down the High Street. I chivalrously swapped baskets, my empty one for her potatoes and onions.

'You haven't changed much,' she said. This simple statement unnerved me almost to the point of saying, as several of Form 5A would surely have done, 'No, apart from this damned false nose.' Prudence constrained me, however.

Far from talking in that worldly nonchalant way that one is led to believe much impresses ladies, my only hope was to try to give the impression that within seconds this social ease would be on display.

'Nor have you.'

In fact, this was untrue. She had changed. It wasn't easy to identify, being an undertone if anything. The flashing smile was not on display, nor the self-assurance and dazzle. How does the moon feel dimmed by the blue splendour of planet Earth and tugged along in its orbit? Certainly on our first acquaintance I had found out just how the moon felt; yet now the roles seemed if not reversed at least more fluid. We walked on and took a left turn.

'I'll go home now,' she said.

'Where's that?'

'Six Walnut Place, where you brought the pheasant.'

'That was years ago.'

'The house hasn't moved, silly.' The moon beamed for a moment.

'But aren't you? I mean if you...'

'Thank you for carrying the groceries.'

Was she living with her parents because she had left her husband, or vice versa? Possibly, but there were hundreds of other reasons: her Mother was ill, her house had burnt down, they had sold up and were about to emigrate. Ninety-nine black slots on the wheel and only one red. It wasn't fair.

How commonplace the circumstances that surround one's crises, or is it just that these decisive moments seem to belong where pigeons are scratching around in the street or someone comes out to pick up the milk bottles or a girl holds a shopping basket. It wasn't as if the lights were going out all over Europe, though for me they soon would be, if, as was quite likely, she got tired of looking at a jellyfish. She mustn't just disappear behind the door. It mustn't happen.

'May I call on you tomorrow?'

It was so Jane Austenish a remark that my brandishing a visiting-card would not have surprised.

'Have you thought about this?' she said.

'For years.'

She smiled: 'Three o'clock then.'

It had to be the turning point, that tide in the affairs of men, which, taken at the flood, leads on to fortune. But something somewhere was very wrong, though exactly what was baffling. In voice and movement she had become unfamiliarly sedate, her air almost one of resignation or indecision. Where was the lustre? I went home and asked Vic, an engineer friend, if he would tune up the car. Throwing out the banana skins could wait until next day.

So far there has been no mention of South Park School. The school was re-organised in 1945 to fulfil the intention of bringing together the brightest eleven-year-old girls of Lincoln and its environs. The city was also served by Christ's Hospital School, once a fee-paying school which my mother had attended, but which thanks to the Butler Education Act aimed to provide, as did South Park, a free and highly academic education for those girls able to pass the entry examination.

For boys the city provided two similar schools, one of which was my alma mater. We both entered our respective establishments on the same day. It was a bold experiment and we were lucky that our young lives so precisely corresponded with it.

Ella and her contemporaries seized their chance avidly and she found herself in a smart brown uniform with orange piping entering what was in no time to become one of the most academic schools in the land. The staff were highly qualified, many with Masters degrees, attracted to this new and exciting development. Into their care came the chosen girls, some seventy or so of them, some older pupils having remained from the previous model. The new girls found wide green playing-fields, a swimming-pool and an imposing head mistress to lead this brave and novel undertaking.

Ella arriving for her first day entered the cloak-room to see her closest friend's new school coat thrown on the floor by a large girl who had decided to have that locker. My love was always the smallest girl in her class but she sprang at the offender and soon the pair were kicking and scratching on the floor.

When she related this, usually as we lay in the dark holding hands, often in some faraway land, she would laugh at how from floor level she saw two long thin shoes, belonging to the headmistress who picked up both of the bedraggled pair.

'What's your name?'

'Ella Burley, Miss.'

'Oh dear, you seem to be in trouble already.'

'Not half as much as I shall be when my mother sees this,' said little Miss

Burley, displaying her new blazer with the pocket torn off. Among the new girls the message resonated. No-one messes with Walnut Place.

Schoolmasters and mistresses alike know that a free spirit, even a turbulent one, usually needs direction; motivation's rarely the problem. Ella was sent to see Miss Higgs, the headmistress, on several occasions but the punishment was always the same: 'You can take my dachshunds out for a walk, Ella, and that will give you a chance to calm down.' Miss Higgs was an Oxford academic and knew potential when she met it.

It was, I'm sure, a fine school and when eventually it published a history of its all too brief existence the title says it all: *Dear South Park.* My dearest girl raced ahead in her studies. Soon she was vying for prizes and for the position of top of her year. She played in hockey, tennis, swimming and chess teams, and was reprimanded for cutting a hole in her beret to allow her pony-tail through. She sped to the top of the Maths and Science classes and was expelled from the choir for tipping over, backwards, a bench of singing girls. Unjustly, according to her, she came second in her final year because the winner's choice of easier subjects let her win. In yet another of those fortuitous ways that one life intersects another the girl who was culpable of so undeservedly coming first became a professor at a Queensland university. She and Ella travelled together to England for a South Park reunion. The professor stayed with us in Adelaide for a couple of nights beforehand and was reminded that her marks for Domestic Science should properly have been discounted. Unabashed the lady found an opportunity to remark good-humouredly that Ella had been lucky to catch a husband like me. It did not go down well with the missus. I didn't mind.

I have already mentioned the little marquetry box containing her fondly remembered items. In it is a letter with her results in the national examination. Six credits, the highest mark, one pass, in English which irked her. From time to time she liked to ask my achievements in the same examination.

Knowing she knew, I would feign forgetfulness. 'You got six credits like me,' she said, 'but three fails. How could anyone fail maths?' Of course she had bounced up onto the stage on Speech Day to collect three prizes.

A sad sequel followed the Speech Day triumph. Her mother was finding herself unable to make ends meet without another wage-earner. Two more years at school and three at university and the budget would never balance. She must leave school.

Miss Higgs in her chauffeured motor-car arrived at Walnut Place. 'Mrs Burley, I will move heaven and earth and get her a place at Oxford.' It was not to be.

VII

The great day, a March Sunday, arrived and the sun shone. It was a nervous morning but Vic had done his stuff. The engine gave a tigerish gurgle-cum-snarl. My youngest brother about to take his Harley Davidson out for a spin was fairly approving.

'Sounds all right but if you get off the drive you'll hear some real power.' My brother Chris was high in my estimation, being not only a steel foundry-man but a confident bare-fist fighter.

'Where's Ann nowadays?' he said. 'Given you the heave-ho?'

'Time for a change,' I said.

'So she did finish it.'

It was clearly pointless practising conversational skills on the drive. Chris was scathingly outspoken and liable to terminate with extreme prejudice whatever he disapproved of. His opinions on my earlier dalliances remain unclear but to my gratification in very little time he and Ella were to become devoted friends.

The previous sentences are prevarications in themselves. It was a nervous time as anything would be better than getting to Lincoln and her not turning up. However the car didn't seize up, or suddenly develop a flat battery, nor did the police intervene with some petty infringement. When I knocked on the door of No.6 her elder sister did not emerge to ask me who I thought I was.

No, she herself emerged, looking lovely but tottering on high spiky heels. 'If we go for a walk, it might be better to wear something more comfortable.'

'Aren't we driving?'

'Well, walking and driving, I thought.'

She went in and emerged with slightly more suitable shoes, and for me a powerful sense of déjà vu.

'Are these suitable enough?'

'I'm sure they are.'

'Well, I'm not wearing Wellington boots!'

It ran through my mind to say that she would look great in such footwear but chose caution. However things improved as she spotted and at once admired my admirable car. It may seem odd that tiny fragments of conversation, even a gesture, remain within recall. Perhaps it is odder that I've forgotten entire years. The rest of the day is hazier but the outline is there.

We drove out into the Lincolnshire countryside that has a charm few other counties understand, driving along lonely roads known to me as a boy with views so long the further landscapes turned blue. We stopped near my uncle's farm and walked, holding hands, through a wood that he owned. I'd played here once upon a time, even camped out with eight-year-old friends. 'That was where my older cousins built a cabin and over there is where the violets grow.' I didn't point out where I'd shot the pheasant.

'I like being with you,' she said.

In later years it became clear to me that the simpler her words the more the depth. The woodland violets were coming into bloom. She picked a handful.

'I'll take these home for my mother.'

During the week my attention had to be with my classes. Not only were the weekdays spent in the classroom, the evenings were filled with sports coaching, then marking books and preparing lessons. It meant working from nine in the morning to ten at night, but if you don't like it then find another job because that's what teaching is. Find a job in the steel foundry.

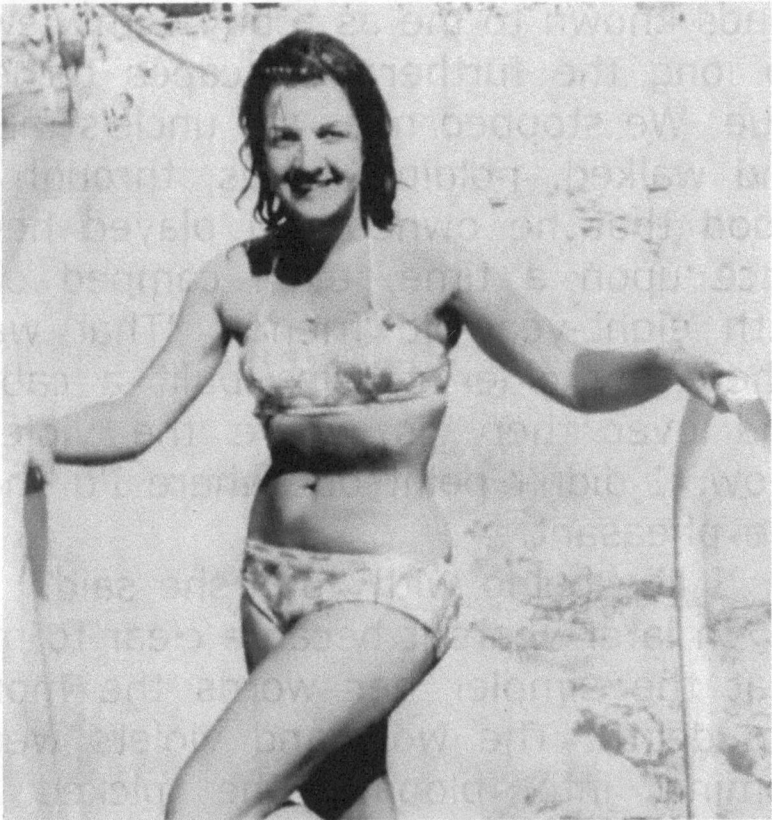

Miss Burley, 1959

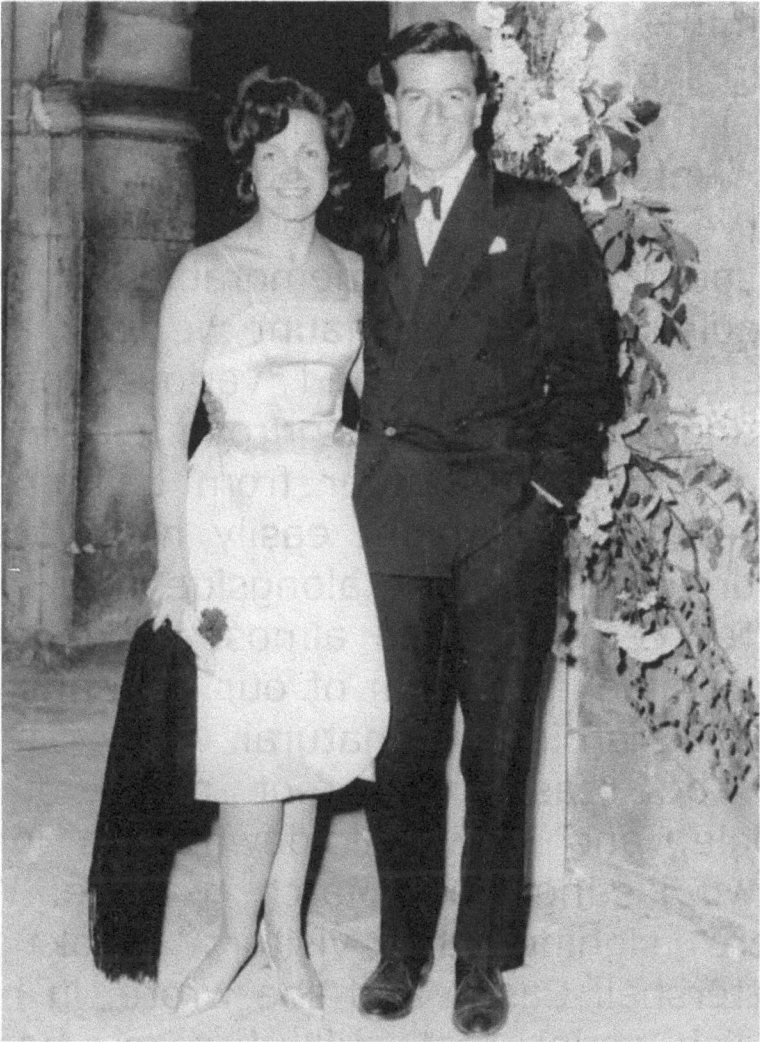

Ella and I at the May Ball, Cambridge, 1962

Saturdays and Sundays were her days and there was never a bad one. Of the details and sequence of our time together I can reproduce only a few. On every weekend in that spring and summer of 1962 the sun shone and we were happy.

I fretted over one thing only: it was an unfamiliar lack of that elan and verve that had made our earlier brief encounter so memorable. She acquiesced in every jaunt we took and there were many and various, often sitting quietly as we drove. In later years this was so far from being the case that she might easily have been a driving instructor alongside me. The latter version would almost have been preferable. The calm of our relationship was disturbingly unnatural.

The reason was not much of a riddle, and slowly it dawned, a long dawn lasting from March to June. We were signing the visitors' book at Tattershall Castle and she wrote, in her stylish script that still stirs my heart when I come across it in her books and letters: Ella Burley.

'Did you keep your own name when you married?' I said, regretting at once walking into this mine-field.

'No.'

'You mean you changed it?'

'Yes, and I don't want to talk about it.'

The matter of her ill-fated marriage was so embedded in self-reproach, repugnance and bitterness that the details took decades to decode, and even then not all of them. Above all she felt a sense of wasted years. She had also during this time almost met a different demon, one that women dread. It would make sense to enclose the days of her first marriage in a section of its own. So wait a while, please.

Tattershall had once belonged to Thomas Cromwell, Chancellor of Henry VIII. Ella was knowledgeable on the Tudor dynasty. She said she found Henry repulsive but Elizabeth admirable, and was happy to justify this historically, adding that the South Park history department 'did the Tudors' every year.

Another time we drove to Fountains Abbey in Yorkshire, largely destroyed by Henry's bully-boys but so hauntingly beautiful even in its dilapidation that in her contempt for Henry she fluffed her hair out and for a few moments resembled her old volatile self as when she had slated me on the phone.

We visited Stowe church, an almost cathedral-like building just north of Lincoln. I wanted to show her the dragon-ship that the Vikings had scratched into the wall of the nave, pretty much as clear today as it was when they sacked the church.

We played golf at Blankney, my home club. She had never played before and alternately missed the ball or hit it a vast distance. 'Silly game,' she said. At the time I had not the slightest idea that she was herself an international sportswoman, not finding this out until about a year later. Had I achieved such a sporting elevation nothing would have stopped me inscribing it on my T-shirts, front and back. In fact our children did give me a T-shirt with the legend 'Hawaii Surf Instructor', which I avoided wearing on the beach lest there be an emergency and desperate people urge me to swim out on a rescue mission. Ella would not have worn it either but would have swum out without hesitation. She swam well and one of my favourite photos of her was taken as she emerged from a pool, as exhilarating and compelling as to the ancients was Venus Anadyomene.

Accidia is an ancient word from the Greek 'akedia' and an interesting concept. It is a form of mental torpor or listlessness. Historically it was most widely noted among solitary ascetics or in monasteries. Where every day is the image of the next with little or no prospect of change it is not difficult to see how one might slip into that condition. Had this accidia, perhaps mild or incipient in form, affected my companion, for if nothing else companions we certainly were.

Several times we walked through Lincoln Cathedral where her father, she told me, had sung as a boy-chorister. A guide told us how before the Reformation the interior walls had been painted red, as some Spanish churches are today. He showed us a small patch of the original red, protected behind a grill. 'Henry VIII again, the vandal', she said disdainfully, more like her old self.

In early May we drove to Cambridge for the day. St John's College was at its best, students and dons in their gowns, the lawns an immaculate velvet and, of course, the 16th century courts, towers and facades as magnificent as ever.

'Which were your rooms?' Billy Davis and I had been lucky having shared splendid rooms and she surveyed them with unfeigned admiration. We strolled on through the courts and over the Bridge of Sighs as punts dawdled beneath, mostly with young men propelling them and girls lolling on cushions.

'Let's go punting'. It was the first time she had proposed an action. Fortunately my punting skills were good, sharpened by many trips on the Cam, not always with attractive girls sadly, more generally with fellow-Johnians who were perfectly ready to push me and one another into the river. Indeed once we spent half an hour diving to recover someone's spectacles from the river-bed.

'Did you ever do any work?' said Ella.

'Course we did, worked like slaves.' A pardonable exaggeration perhaps, soon dismissed.

'Rubbish,' she said.

We hired a punt and decorously manoeuvred up-river past the spectacle of Trinity and Kings, under the Mathematical Bridge and moored at the Garden House Hotel to drink champagne.

'I wish I'd gone to Cambridge.'

'You'd have got a first in Maths.'

'Perhaps. Did you take other girls on the river?'

'Dozens.'

'Where are they now?'

'*Ou sont les neiges d'antan?*' Too easy a line for a South Park girl.

'Melted away like the snow have they? Yes, well, on second thoughts I will have another champagne.'

Would life always be as good as this? Why not? Cambridge wouldn't run away. I hoped she wouldn't. Later she bestowed a kiss, soft as a moth's wings. Softer than a butterfly.

On went the summer unclouded. My Sussex acquaintances asked me to play cricket at Eastbourne. She watched from the pavilion balcony and runs came again. Was the wheel ever to deliver black? In the far future we were to go years without a red. After the game the

Austin Healey purred across the spaciousness of the South Downs.

'Look down there,' I said. 'That's where Duke William and the Normans came ashore, and not far east of here Julius Caesar and the Romans landed.'

We stopped for the night at a little village called Beeding.

'Two rooms,' she said. 'There's no rush.'

'Nothing was further from my mind.'

'I am married, you know.'

'I couldn't care less about that.' It changes one's perspectives, the hands around the throat.

'I know,' she said. 'So long as you care about me.'

Next day, being no distance from Brighton, we visited the Royal Pavilion. It is an extravaganza of a place, Indian-Moghul outside with a more or less Chinese interior, in all a dilettante opulence reflective of the Prince Regent himself. Though finding it self-indulgent I enjoyed visiting and had done so several times while teaching at Shoreham. Ella's reaction was, though I had no previous reason to expect this, to head for the Great Kitchen to commiserate with the long-gone kitchen maids who once earned a derisory wage for nurturing the hedonism of the Prince, later George IV, and his sycophantic court. On the way home she revealed that her mother had worked 'downstairs' in a nabob's mansion in Gloucestershire, where usefully she had learnt to prepare a pheasant.

She had revelled in the visit to Cambridge so we did it again. This time we planned a punting trip further up the river to Grantchester, a pleasant university tradition.

'Grantchester,' she said. 'I've heard of it somewhere.'

Punting there took quite some time but the banks were bedecked with flowers, the air scented by lime-trees and everywhere butterflies zigzagging. She quietly scrutinised other ladies whom we passed or were passed by but was clearly satisfied with her choice of a green and white dress. How could I forget the willows and the river eddies swirling?

Footfalls echo in the memory

*Down the passage which we did
not take
Towards the door we never opened
Into the rose garden.*

Except we did open it and went through it together. What we didn't know was what came after the rose garden.

We paddled into the shallows and walked to the tea-garden. It must have had roses. Ella surprised me by suddenly reciting from Rupert Brooke's poem *Grantchester:*

*Stands the church clock at ten to three,
And is there honey still for tea?*

She knew it from school. Of course there was honey and tea and scones. She said 'I love this.'

The accidia was still there. Every allusion, every blind alley, traced back to her marriage. In what entrapment had she found herself? I couldn't ask and she wouldn't say other than once to mention his name: Carter.

'His name, not mine,' she added spikily.

My next proposition prospered from the start. Tickets for the Royal Shakespeare Theatre in Stratford-upon-Avon: Friday night *The Tempest,* Saturday afternoon *Midsummer Night's Dream.* She came in a handsome new coat, a vivid red colour. What could go wrong? She was by nature extremely careful with money but had clearly lashed out for the occasion.

The Tempest refers to the storm which wrecked a ship full of interesting characters on the recently-discovered island of Bermuda. Shakespeare tackles one of his age's great problems – the relation between the autochthons of the New World and their European conquerors: an interaction which vexes Australia today. The primitive Caliban who once owned the island is a stunningly original creation, and though clearly dangerous, amoral and brutish still touched Ella's soft heart when he woke to find his island taken from him and he 'cried to dream again', as did I in the then distant future.

The next afternoon was *Midsummer Night's Dream,* her favourite play, in which years later our daughter was to take the role of Titania. I have seen a great many of Shakespeare's plays but never one so brilliant, so light-hearted, so exuberant as we saw that afternoon. My girl, though mildly scandalised that Titania was bewitched into sleeping with a donkey, was almost hysterical with laughter at the antics of the rustics, notably Bottom the weaver. As we drove back to Lincoln she was buoyant, animated and talked non-stop. I was glad, and why not? She was the brightest of the bright and Shakespeare was her heritage.

'Is it true?' she said. 'You know: "We are such stuff as dreams are made on, and our little life is rounded with a sleep."'

'We'll find out together,' I said.

As a little girl she had joined Mrs Maclean's Concert Party. This was a well-known institution and a remarkably professional one. They set up quite a number of concerts, mostly with singers and dancers, but also skits and sketches and solo acts. The performers were children and usually quite young. They appeared once in the village hall of my own village and quite possibly I may have seen the Party's leading tap-dancer for this was her speciality, though not exclusively so. Once with me in Galway she hopped up onto the stage, smoothly integrating into a line of Irish dancers, then doing exactly the same in Spain, joining into a strange slow pastoral dance in the market square in a remote pueblo in Navarre. When asked what she as a girl had aspired to become she would say nostalgically, 'A chorus girl'.

In truth she was a virtuoso. Trying to find a gap in her repertoire I recall quizzing her: Can you dance the bossa nova? Yes. Cha cha? Yes. Flamenco? Yes, I like that. Polka? Yes. Rumba? Of course, who can't? Tango? That's my second favourite. What's your favourite then? Rock and roll – it keeps my weight down.

I proffered a few implausible possibilities: Hula-hula? I would if I had a grass skirt. Charleston? Yes, it's nice. Can-can? Probably not if people were watching. She boasted that she'd never refused a request to dance, though that didn't commit her to continuing if there was what she called funny stuff.

So who was her favourite partner? Without hesitation she said, 'Hugh'.

'Oh, you mean Hugh Halket?' It made some sort of sense. Hugh was a realistic candidate whom we both knew well, lively, good company and the right credentials, being from Lime Grove.

'Hugh?' said Ella. Or was it 'Who?' or even 'Huw'. Maybe Halket was Welsh.

'Is Hugh your favourite dancing partner?'

'Who? Hugh?' she giggled at this off-the-cuff owl noise. 'No, you, you!'

'Good heavens. I'm no good.'

'You're OK, unless the dance ends in a vowel. Also you don't pump my arm up and down or get too close.'

'I could if...'

'Later, later,' she said. Though occasionally she would pretend for a moment to be risqué she would never do it outside the charmed circle of the two of us. In truth she was modest and without an atom of coarseness or vulgarity. It was what made her so endearing. Nothing could subvert her natural virtue. Or so I thought then.

It was now June, therefore time for the Cambridge May Balls. St John's always threw a good show though tickets weren't easily come by. The rooms on what had been our staircase, I First Court, were the domain of Mrs Driver, our bedder, the term referring to a mix of bed-making and generally preventing us from existing in layers of filth or even layers of sloth. Mrs D was an iron lady long before Mrs Thatcher, but she had a soft spot for Billy Davis my room-mate and even at times for me. 'You've been climbing in again, Mr Roe and Mr Davis. You'll do yourselves a mischief on those spikes.' Chapel Court's spiked railings were twelve feet high and a tough climb in the dark but a convenient entry-point when the College locked itself up. Mrs Driver was often the matriarch and major-domo of the Ball, in charge of supper and drinks. She posted the tickets when called upon.

When Ella heard of this she announced she would take a half day off work. My reassurance that we could set off at 5.30pm and easily get there was brushed off, on the grounds that five hours preparation would still mean rushing it. As it turned out the only rush was caused by my fetching the heel off my shoe, done while kicking about with the lads in the playground at lunch-time. This meant wearing brown suede shoes, my only other footwear apart from football boots. I had some mad idea about buying a pair on the way, though the A1 motorway would have had few shoe shops. Maybe no-one would notice.

When collected Ella certainly noticed and, adopting the bearing of an over-loaded Mother Superior, went inside and borrowed her brother's shoes for me. She was wearing her newish red coat, tightly buttoned and carrying her shoes in a paper bag along with a silk stole, the girls in the office having all chipped in. Clearly her outfit was to be a secret.

'What will the Ball be like?'

'OK,' I said soothingly.

'If it's just OK, we'll go back so I can get sandals and a cardigan.'

We arrived. She darted into the ladies' room and some time passed. When she emerged I was transfixed.

Her dress was ice-floe blue, the colours sliding into one another, her evening bag and shoes, none of which items I had been allowed to see, an exact match. Her hair was sunset red. She was utterly beautiful. This all sounds pretty adolescent but you've got to call it how it is. Anyway it's the stark truth and my sorrow was and is not having the imagination to find the words to enshrine that truth. Several girls nearby turned and went back for more lipstick or something.

We walked into the Great Hall where a dance band so famous I'm unable to recall its name was playing. Mrs Driver, doing a duchess impersonation, put into Ella's hand a red rose and a dance card. The card is inevitably in her marquetry box.

'Look,' she said. 'I've never had one before. I'm going to fill it all in.'

'Well, leave me a space somewhere. Remember there'll be about six or seven other bands around the College courts.' There were: a jazz band, a string ensemble, a rock band, a Caribbean steel band, even a group calling themselves a skiffle band. Probably there were others. Maybe even Bottom the weaver who had a reasonable good ear for music and played the tongs and bones.

We managed a decorous waltz. A friend of mine Jack Willis asked her to dance. She wrote his name on her card for later. When it came it was a foot-stamping eye-catching paso doble.

'Olé, who is she?' said Jack. 'I'm going to ask her for every dance.'

'What about your partner?'

'Will you dance with her?'

'No, Jack, no. You dance with the one what brung you.'

Mrs Driver came over with champagne and caviar. 'Goodness me,' she whispered. 'Where did you find her?'

'In a tax office, Mrs D.'

Ella said, 'I do like caviar.'

From somewhere I found a ditty:

Caviar's the roe of a virgin sturgeon,
A sturgeon's a very rare fish,
Not every sturgeon's a virgin sturgeon
So caviar's a very rare dish.

Mrs Driver brought more champagne and asked fondly: 'Have you seen Mr Davis lately?'

'No I haven't.' How could I? Billy Davis was dead, the first of the singers in the pub to go. Undermined by melancholia he ended his own life. It shocked me, the condition seeming flimsy, a sort of fragility or loneliness but nothing fatal. Maybe it was a daemon with a respectable 'a'. I thought of myself as lucky but my friends' luck was being siphoned off. Tom and Billy had been close to me and Ella was close. I didn't like the sequence, or the semblance of a sequence, and the sequel didn't bear thinking of.

It was 8am when we reached Lincoln with a class waiting to be taught in Cleethorpes at 8.45. It would mean teaching in a dinner jacket which would entertain the boys more used to my customary tatty sports coat. As it turned out none of their ribbing mattered.

The car drew up outside Walnut Place and we got out and walked to the door. The listlessness of her earlier months had gradually faded away and after that night never came back. Like a rainbow's arch the future beckoned us to walk through it.

You see as Ella stood poised to go in she turned and said, 'Do you love me?' and since the question's difficulty fell into the category of which letter is next in the alphabet after A, I said, 'Yes, of course I do,' which was pretty much what she knew anyway. 'Good,' she said. 'I love you.' In my heart there was a certainty that she meant it. Thank heaven I was able to avoid some Wildean remark to the effect that the only thing worse than falling in love was not falling in love. With the benefit of hindsight it might have been not completely untrue to say we hardly knew one another for she had a depth and subtlety of character that our renewed acquaintance of about four or five months, a sort of idyllic holiday, was far too short and starry-eyed for me to grasp. What I did grasp with total certainty was my happiness whenever we were together and with a sort of disbelief that it could be happening. What did the most beautiful and delightful girl imaginable think she was doing saying that she loved me?

But her words were too elemental for doubt. It's an interesting word, elemental, composed of the elements of earth, air, fire and water, a force of nature, which, of course, is what love is. But it has a dark side, as an elemental may be also a psychic occult manifestation such as the one that in the twilight of our lives was so freakishly hurtful. The creature that savaged me in my dream was an elemental too, a psychic creature if ever there was one.

VIII

With total clarity, I recall moments in the last months of Ella's life, when I despaired of ever hearing it again, she said 'I love you' with all the certitude and trust as she had on that very morning after the Ball, and despite our mutual distress those words from an eighty-year-old lady thrilled and invigorated me and somewhere the demon in its pomp flinched. It flinched just as Apollyon had cowered away when Christian on his hands and knees fought back saying, 'Nay, in all these things we are more than conquerors through Him that loved us'. Christian was inclined to rhetoric at critical moments and only just avoids it here, but 'I love you' isn't rhetoric at all, whether it's Christ's love or that of a humble married couple. Anyway our spectre, like the monstrous Apollyon, would certainly interpret it as defiance. As indeed it was. The demon hurt her cruelly, but it never broke her.

The days of August and September 1962 moved on gently though autumnally. It'll turn out all right in the end whenever we get round to thinking about it. This was not unlike my usual attitude to crises but utterly unlike Ella's. To her a crisis was a call for action or a call for me to do something about it whichever suited her, nor would she be put off by being informed there was no need to panic like the Gadarene swine. When she did take action that autumn it was physical and the operation accelerated. The major reason for our lotos-eating idyll of that summer was her unreadiness even to discuss her marriage or any legal, ethical, moral or practical consequences of its existence. However when she did bring herself to speak about it, gradually and reluctantly releasing information over several years, one could only sympathise with her reticence.

The late summer months were the time of the informal cricket clubs, a number of whom I'd played for or against. The lively Suffolk Clergymen CC had often visited St John's; at Eastbourne I'd played with the Sussex Martlets and now there was an invitation to be one of the Lincolnshire

Ramblers to play at Elsham village. It's a nice place, tucked under the Wolds in the north of the county, and there that afternoon we played village cricket at its most enjoyable, quietly friendly while properly competitive as no doubt the game had always been played there. Wives and girlfriends sat on deck-chairs and came in for tea and strawberries. It was dusk when we finished and owls were calling as we drove through the warm evening with the hood back. The street-lamps were on as we wound through the small market-town of Brigg.

Ella said, 'Stop here.'

'Why?'

'Because I don't want to go home.'

For a moment I was perplexed and then she giggled. Maybe she blushed but it was hard to tell in the twilight.

As I mentioned earlier my mother was an accomplished pianist. As a small boy, when not driven out as a distraction, it was intriguing to sit with her as she practised or rehearsed or simply amused herself playing, as D.H. Lawrence knew:

A child sitting under the piano, in
the boom of the tingling strings
And pressing the small poised feet
of a mother who smiles as she
sings.

The sequence rarely varied. First came the scales, rippled through with a flawless and awesome dexterity. Then usually came Bach and Mozart. 'Sonata for Clavier and Violin' she would say. 'Allegro, then Andante, then Allegretto gracioso.' Finally came what was to me the highlight, when playing entirely for fun she would play negro spirituals and amuse herself by calling out the tempo and after a few moments change abruptly in mid-piece: 'Adagio' she would say, then 'Crescendo, Vivamenta, Amorosa, Forte' and 'Generoso' which seemed to mean wild and was an especial favourite, suiting her dark and sultry good looks. Of the spirituals themselves only one title remains 'Camptown Races' and the memorable lines:

Well I came down there with my
hat caved in, doo-dah, doo-dah,

Oh, I'll go back home with my
pocket full of tin, doo-dah, doo-dah
day.

If you are wondering why this little diversion on musical tempos, I'll explain. That eventually we should make love was likely enough but that she, not I, should decide the moment seemed to me the only course leading to long-term happiness. In this regard her ill-fated marriage though kept largely hidden from me had apparently been without anything, or anything significant, of the passion, the imagination and magnetism of love. To know passion is to live. There are subsidiary passions: music, cricket, breeding guinea-pigs, trainspotting. They may well enliven life, but they pale before the grand passion. I'm sure (these aren't my words but the author escapes me) that for many people knowing a grand passion is about as likely as composing a Grand Opera, and sadly that's the way the wheel spins.

But she had the utmost possession of my heart and it would be ever thus. One could only hope it was reciprocal.

Certainly it seemed so that night and for many years to come. She was a passionate lover and made my previous inadequate dalliances seem not tawdry for they weren't, but trifling. That's all, except that the musical tempos are not after all irrelevant. If her love-making was restricted to two terms only they would be in turn: *allegro,* merry and bright, and *generoso,* generous and with abandon. What the musical term is for dream-like eludes me.

A couple of weeks later she asked me to drive her over to the house of her marriage. It was in a pleasant though rather anonymous residential part of the city, identical semi-detached houses either side of a wide road, with smallish but well-tended gardens though most without garages. Not far off was an attractive park with a sizable lake, and further on some hard tennis courts. Cars were lined along the edge of the road. We had to park some way away and walk towards her house.

'Do you own a car?' I asked.

'That's going to be a problem.'

'What's the problem?'

'Well, who actually owns it?'

This remained a mystery for a while as a man in a khaki raincoat seemed to be trailing along behind us. He seemed slightly familiar.

'Do you know him?'

She shrugged, was edgy and began to walk faster. By now I was starting to mind-read a little, one of those skills that married couples practise to perfection.

'I'll say hello to him,' I said, taking a step in that direction.

She grabbed my arm: 'No, no, don't. It doesn't matter.'

'You obviously know who he is.'

'Yes. He's a private detective. He's been following us around lately.'

'Let me discourage him.'

'No, no, no.'

'Verbally deter him?'

'No.'

'You should let me look after you.'

I walked towards the man in the raincoat, who in turn walked away. After about a hundred yards with the distance closing between us he stopped and got into a car. I rapped on the window and gestured to him to open it. He shook his head. I tried the door. It was locked. There was some rubble on a nearby building-site so I fetched a half-brick and tapped it on the windshield. He looked away so I gave the door a tap, making a clanging noise and removing some paint. He wound the window down about three inches and said, 'What do you want?'

'I'd just like to talk to you.'

'You want to mind your own business.'

Let me pause (not that there was any let-up at the time) to remark that throughout my life whenever I met that particular phrase it generally referred to staying out of some altercation in which I wished and had every right to be very much involved. The red mist that now and again corroded my better judgement in those days was starting to swirl and the brick seemed to want to join in. But the man was much smaller than I was and probably thirty years older. He seemed to have been recommended by a down-at-heel casting agency for a cameo appearance as a washed-out agent.

'Listen! Forget you ever heard of Ella. She is the innocent party here. I'll take care of it. You are not needed. Use what passes as your brain and do not get involved!'

Presumably he wished to leave as the motor started. I pushed the brick in through the window and it dropped on his lap, perfectly duplicating in reverse a similar event about four years later – another coincidence for a lengthening list.

I walked back to Ella. 'I saw the brick,' she said.

'Did you?'

We were both quiet, she for her own reasons, leaving me to feel remorseful for my hectoring behaviour. There had been an occasion about the age of fourteen when I'd hit my classmate, Micky Gent, on the head with a half-brick in a fight that got out of hand. I remember it vividly, not so much for my cretinous action as for the confrontation afterwards between my mother and Micky's when the latter came knocking on the door. Mum forgot her lady of the manor demeanour and met Mrs Gent as equals, or rather as screeching viragos, particularly after Mrs Gent seemed to regard Mum's describing it as 'boyish high-jinks' as understating the case.

My father, had he been at home, would have been placatory and understanding and probably asked the lady in for a cup of tea, but that's not how the female of the species operates. In adult life I met Micky a couple of times and felt no hard feelings. He had clearly neither forgotten nor forgiven which was very un-christian of him. The scar was still visible on his hairline.

It occurred to me to ask Ella how long we had been under observation.

'Well, several days, off and on.'

'I didn't notice.'

'Didn't you? Really?' She laughed rather as if I had failed to notice one of those princely progresses of three thousand elephants carrying the Maharajah of Mysore, a multitude of followers and the opulence of his seraglio to the Durbar with the Raj, just behind us, making its majestic way through Lincoln's streets, but by me unnoticed.

'Forget the elephants,' I said, briefly on a more exotic planet, 'and let's sort this business out.'

'High time, because I think I'm pregnant.'

When one is recreating the past, back from across fifty years or so, it is not usually possible to recall precise conversations. Though occasionally this can be done, actions are much simpler to revivify, often exactly. Nevertheless her announcement was certainly a conversation stopper and I'm sure I've remembered that particular remark word for word. Even the elephants faded away as our world re-aligned itself.

We went back to her mother's house for a consultation and the formation of a plan. As I've said an Ella plan and my plan were very different aspirations. Hers, it seemed to me, was over-tolerant and charitable. Mine she described as the damage an unimaginative bull could do when loose in a china-shop. Here's where the Algeciras incident worked as an allegory. Do something quick, you get lucky, whoever hesitates gets hurt and deserves it, whether in Spain or Lincoln. It probably works half the time, but I believed in it then.

There was no-one at home at 6 Walnut Place but us, so we sat at the kitchen table and I proposed to her. There were tears and protests that without her pregnancy it would never have happened. She cheered up when told that she must surely have known perfectly well she was my beloved and always had been and did she intend to consent or just dither around.

After a bit more dithering she did consent and that was that. The next item was when. The month was October, the date about the 20th. There was the problem of where to live, both geographically and specifically. The first was easy, the second harder but Ella wished to take on that problem herself and find somewhere in the imposing conurbation of Grimsby and Cleethorpes.

We decided on early January, Saturday the third, with a honeymoon before school started which would be about the twelfth of that month. Her mother could fix up the details of the wedding day. The finances we'd cope with somehow or more accurately she would. Thus far it was not so difficult but it assumed that she would be divorced by January. That needed to be hastened, particularly as nothing much had happened so far other than the business of the agent in the khaki raincoat.

'Does your husband want a divorce?'

'Yes, of course. But he wants to divorce me on the grounds of my adultery and then keep the house and car and so on.'

Remember this was 1962 and the divorce laws were about as inequitable as equity can get.

'Have you got a key to the house? Yes? Then go round there, bring all your personal belongings and store them in your bedroom.' Ella's two sisters had married and moved out so there was some unaccustomed space.

'So he gets nearly everything? Is that your plan?'

'I don't care. Forget things like chairs and pots and pans. We'll start from scratch. Every other married couple does.'

'Do I get an engagement ring?'

'Yes, next weekend. I'll win you one at Wonderland.'

'Will you win me a wedding ring too?'

'I can only try. You can sometimes fish one out with those crane things.'

'Good. I got rid of his ring ages ago. I should have thrown it in the Witham.' The Witham was Lincoln's turgid river flowing through the city and on to sluice into the muddy waters of the Wash.

'When did you do that?'

'Oh, after about four or five months.'

Thus the first information of her previous marriage was divulged. For the rest one must wait. There was still plenty to do and it wasn't going to get any easier.

We were blissfully happy that spring and summer, even part of the way into autumn, but such a state of mind only exists undisturbed when outside daily reality.

'Human kind cannot bear very much reality.' T.S. Eliot got it absolutely right, yet amazingly love can survive reality, a little bruised perhaps, but that comes with the adventure. Anyway the time had come for us to emerge and tackle as a couple the legal and familial problems ahead. One Everest-like challenge was that my mother, who had yet to meet Ella, was not going to take kindly to a married woman or premature pregnancy or the adultery business.

To see how it all untangled, or at least to what extent it untangled, it might help to look at some of the protagonists, excluding Ella and myself, as you're already acquainted with us. The Burley family were either expert at concealing opinion or essentially not bothered. Her father was fond of her and protective but somehow excluded from the family in a way difficult to understand. Partly no doubt this was due to his army life isolating him in barracks or overseas, and even after retirement he had worked as Head of Security at Scampton, the famous airfield of the Dambusters. He was reclusive enough for me only to have met him once. He died in the second year of our marriage. Ella often told me of a frightening occasion when she was walking home, as so often, from the Co-op Ballroom late at night and was pursued by a man. She took off her shoes and fled through the dark, rushing into the family room to find her father there. The chasing man entered their small yard and actually peered in the window. Mr Burley rose, went outside and came back.

'Has he gone?' asked our girl.

'Not yet,' said her father. After an hour the man was still lying in the yard. 'Stop looking out the window and go to bed. He'll be gone in the morning.' As he was. I'm mildly surprised that her father didn't dish out similar treatment to her first husband and probably would have done had he known the truth of the relationship.

Mrs Burley was a most capable lady. She came from Bath and had clearly been a striking and handsome lady who after six children had put on weight. She managed everything, not only her own offspring and household but, as far as one could tell, supervising at least twenty other nearby families and any number of pensioners. She was a source of urban know-how, doing everything from playing in the local pub's darts team to delivering innumerable babies. She became my ally and friend. I thought Ella, of all the children, resembled her most closely.

The others played only small parts. George the oldest ran a business, played golf and had clearly left Walnut Place. Betty, the lady in curlers, regarded me, though I cannot think why, as a privileged wealthy playboy who would seduce and rapidly abandon her sister. It would be Tess of the d'Urbervilles all over again. Or indeed Little Nell. She gave the impression Ella should persevere in her hopeless marriage, though would only have done so herself if allowed to be overbearing and shrewish. The second and younger sister I liked a lot. Sadly a different demon scarred her life. The youngest sibling, Dave, was admirable in every way, an upright young man who later became a good friend.

My own family were much more volatile, parents and children being all unalike, all with centrifugal opinions and lifestyles, along for that matter with two outspoken grannies. The family conference, when it came, was incendiary. The most rational members were my father and my brother Chris, who took the attitude of interested but uncommitted bystanders, forgoing cries of moral uprightness. My parents were an unusual though utterly devoted couple. My father had lost his father at the age of fourteen and being unable to inherit the family business set out to work as a builder's labourer, though retaining a substantial expanse of meadows and arable land. By 1940 he was a master-builder and then spent the next five years in the army, campaigning in North Africa, Sicily, Italy and Norway. He had Viking blood in him, tall blue-eyed and handsome, a stoical and honourable man. There were several mutual visits involving families he had helped to liberate, and I recall both Norwegians and Algerian *pieds-noirs* staying with us and my parents with them. His attitude was if it doesn't kill you it makes you stronger and, like me, he believed in luck. As an impoverished young brickie he bet every penny he could muster on April the Fifth (i.e. a horse not that date) to win the Derby, April the fifth being my mother's birthday. It romped home, winning him so much money that my mother's mother smiled upon him and agreed to part with her daughter.

My mother, I knew for certain, was going to kick up a monumental fuss. She had been brought up in Heighington House, and was the only survivor of three daughters, two dying as teenagers. She was used to the big splendid house in which I spent my first five years and to its maids, nannies, cooks and skivvies of one sort or another. When my father came home from the war they bought a house with the proceeds earned by April the Fifth. Mum was a well-known pianist but had many interests. She was widely travelled, inclined to go off to concerts in Vienna and showed no concern when in Rhodesia our car was buffeted by elephants. She loved gardening and plants and was herself a botanist. Walking with her across a meadow one was regaled with the grasses' identities: timothy grass, Yorkshire fog, yellow oat-grass, fox-tail. I used to know them once. She forgave my siblings most things and me very little. I was the first-born and must lead the way and certainly not get entangled with an adventuress. This term was so incongruous it was hardly worth pointing out that it was an unusual adventuress who coveted my bank account which was, as usual, deeply in the red. Nothing wrong with red, if you spend bravely: vide the Austen Healey.

The family conference was a sparky affair. There seemed several agendas in play apart from the obvious angst. General opinion was that my attitude to being named as the guilty party, indisputably and undisputed, was far too nonchalant. In fact I couldn't care less and made it known. Unfortunately the local newspaper's policy was to treat divorces as world-shaking news, the publicity inflaming my mother's wrath, she quickly seeing through my subterfuge of giving my address as 'of Burnham-on-Crouch'. She also saw through an incident a week before when with my car being serviced I had cycled into Lincoln and on the way home about midnight I'd been charged with the heinous crime of riding a bike without lights on a completely deserted country road. This time, totally jacked off, I'd given my name as Micky Jent, with a

'J', of Burnham-on-Crouch. This key misdemeanour had featured prominently in the same newspaper, causing one of my friends to write to the paper (and get his letter published) purporting to be puzzled by the authorities' inaction faced with a migrant crime wave. Happy days. I wish they'd come back.

When in our conference the furor broke around my head I tried to ignore the disparagement or play it down but after about twenty minutes (how accommodating to accept it that long) my patience evaporated. It was time for the Algeciras response which consisted of exploding in a rage, to me at least well-justified, and pointing out that Ella was now my fiancée, would shortly be my wife, and that was exactly how it was going to be and unless she was invited around for tea at the weekend and was treated kindly and respectfully then we'd better all shake hands and say farewell for the foreseeable future.

The tea-party was not quite as historically significant as the Boston Tea-party but both had their moments. My mother kept herself at a distance and made her displeasure known by providing not her usual haute cuisine but, not quite able to shake off her upbringing, sending out cucumber sandwiches into the garden. My father, of course, was his honourable self and my other brother Geoff, who was an ingrained mischief-maker, fortunately had to leave early. Ella, it hardly needs saying, was ultra-polite and pleasant. She was anyway in my father's good books for her skills with the company's tax, plus her extra-curricular labour in clearing up my financial confusion and in no time he was won over, particularly by her admiring his dog, a much-pampered whippet. Even she would not have found the slightest redeeming feature in my sister's dog, which was that afternoon kept locked in the garage, it having previous form. This hound of Hades had a month or so earlier attacked me as I came through the garden gate, torn the sleeve off an expensive coat and bitten deep into my arm. In a frenzy of pain and shock I had beaten it against the garden wall, little expecting to be threatened by my sister with the RSPCA as I left to get help with injections against rabies.

Again, as so often, the future had a little quirk up its sleeve. On the sad day that we buried my love's ashes my sister gave me our father's deed-box. Her dog, thank heaven, had by this time gone to meet its maker. The box was familiar but empty except for a roll of undeveloped film. The Adelaide photo shop did a good job as the film was fifty-four years old. Most pictures were of Cambridge but there were four, much treasured, of Ella at the tea-party. It was like being given the Koh-i-noor diamond. But better.

IX

The divorce went through without any of the concerned parties having to meet. In fact my acquaintance with her first husband did not exist other than, I suppose, having seen the photograph in the newspaper's office-window. There remained only for Ella to leave the Tax Office after twelve years employment there and acquiring accommodation somewhere in or near Grimsby.

In her time at the Tax Office she had unsurprisingly risen from most junior office-girl charged with making tea to a very senior position. Had romance not intervened she would have risen high in her, or almost any, profession. She had been marked for promotion and placed at Leeds University for a year, emerging with a Diploma in Finance. She had enjoyed her studies and had lodged with a Jewish family. They were, she said, so kind that she always supported Israel in its various skirmishes with the Arab world. In fact, as Miss Higgs her headmistress had observed, she had an unusually clear and orderly mind. Mathematics came easily to her and of its branches she was fondest of geometry. Where her talents might have taken her remains an enigma but there was a very clear sign. About a year before we became re-acquainted she took the Civil Service examination. It is an examination designed to identify the type of mind able to cope with the pressures and demands of administering a modern state. The civil servants who operate the great departments of state in Britain diversify into twenty-three professional areas and almost certainly her skills would have placed her in one of either Economics or Finance. So how did she fare in her examination? With distinction, of course, placing sixteenth. She was unsure of the number of examinees and could only surmise at several thousands. It was just as well I'd met her with her onions and potatoes or she would have been bound for London to become a protégée of Sir Humphrey Appleby of *Yes Minister* fame, or his like, which from my point of view would have been a thoroughly bad thing.

When asked if she regretted the path she didn't take she said several times and emphatically: 'I wanted a family and children and I thought it was never going to happen.' So no regrets at all.

> Two roads diverged in a yellow wood,
> And sorry I could not travel both
> And be one traveller, long I stood
> And looked down one as far as I could
> To where it bent in the undergrowth;
> Then took the other...

> I shall be telling this with a sigh
> Somewhere ages and ages hence:
> Two roads diverged in a wood and I–
> I took the one less travelled by,
> And that has made all the difference.

She would talk freely of her Tax Office days, of her many friends there and of our meeting on the road less travelled. She liked to discuss geometry and would remind me of how the great

Greek philosophers were fascinated by its nature: Pythagoras, Euclid, Archimedes to name only a few. She had been well taught. Spacial relationships came easily to her and twenty years later she would take a degree using that special gift. As if I could forget her standing there in her academic gown and mortar-board.

When discussing her Tax Office days she occasionally used words that meant nothing to me. There was, for instance, what sounded like a special linguistic group: Aslackoe, which she often mentioned and what sounded like its relations, Wraggoe and Langoe among others. Eventually it was explained, though she enjoyed using this insider jargon. Exasperated by my referring to it as gobbledegook (a word that appealed to me and still does) she accused me of ignorance and insensitivity, traits displayed by me on meeting the raincoat man. 'QED' she would say, triumphantly using her geometrical insider jargon.

When the facts about Aslackoe came out it fascinated me. The Tax Office used the terms to allocate parts of the county to their officers. Aslackoe, Ella's speciality, covered the area around the small town of Gainsborough. The mystifying words were all areas of Lincolnshire. Langoe, for instance, covered the area of Heighington. My History studies started to respond. These were the wapentakes, the weapon councils of the distant past before the Norman Conquest. Most other counties knew these administrative units as 'hundreds', but the Danelaw, of which Lincolnshire was part, stubbornly hung onto wapentakes. No other county was as intractable and resistant to Norman occupation as Lincolnshire and under the leadership of Hereward the Wake the fenlanders had fought on until 1072, six years after William's victory at Hastings. The only places outside Britain still to use 'hundreds' are a few of the oldest states of the USA and, amazingly, South Australia. If you don't believe me look it up on Google. Good for SA, though sad that they don't use wapentakes.

This odd little facet of history appealed to both of us. She loved her country and her county, as did I.

England meant much to her. She was a fully paid-up royalist with no time for Oliver Cromwell, particularly as his troopers had stabled their horses in Lincoln Cathedral and shot out the windows. She was politically right-wing, always voting Conservative, rationalising this on the grounds that she was voting for Winston Churchill. Certain nationalities were regarded coldly, though how they had offended was not always clear. West Indians were one such group and Arabs, a generic term covering plenty of nations, another. A special corner of hell was reserved for Nazis.

Having failed in Wonderland's arcades I bought her an engagement ring. She liked rings and, on what seemed to be appropriate occasions, particularly in later life, her fingers would flash with diamonds. By now she had, or said she had, adopted my view that the divorce was a legal triviality and a brisk interview with some lawyer or other established her legal freedom. 'A pity they wouldn't give me back those years,' she said stoically.

The wedding day approached and arrived without fanfare. She had somehow done wonders with our marital accommodation, both in finding and furnishing it. It was the ground floor of a large house in Grimsby, placed looking onto People's Park which sounded like, but wasn't, a place in Stalingrad full of brutalist Bolshevik statuary. There were several spacious rooms and in no time she had decorated and furnished them. Curtains and carpets came flying in. My parents, who didn't really know Ella, had provided furniture for the biggest room in order to avoid us living in penniless squalor. This included a stylish escritoire with pigeon holes which she seized upon as her administrative centre. Fortunately the County Council had given her a leaving bonus and this and a little money she had saved enabled her to work wonders with our new home. As she said afterwards, many times, she would have been more economical with these wonders had she known the size of my overdraft, which had almost become a bottomless pit after I'd bought her a wedding ring that Croesus would have admired.

Our landlord, a jovial business-man, behaved as if mesmerised by my wife-to-be and gave us the use of the garage and the garden and charged a minimal rent. My colleagues at school gave us a splendid dinner service. How kind people were! Amazing. My days in dubious lodgings would soon be a thing of the past.

Mrs Burley, and I never addressed her by any other name, ran the wedding. It began with another lawyer in another dusty room formalising the marriage vows. The place, the occasion, have faded away except for the words 'a solemn and binding contract'. They stuck in my head and we stuck by them. Then we gathered for the reception at the White Hart Hotel, a pleasant though rather starchy establishment close to Lincoln's great Norman cathedral. Gathering there was less straightforward than it sounds as it was snowing heavily and my new sister-in-law Rhonda broke the later conversational ice by being unable to stop as her car slid helplessly and spectacularly into another vehicle stationary at traffic lights.

The two families, as at all weddings I've attended, took a little time to unthaw and work out which tribe if any had made an aggregate gain from the marriage. How things unfold in the later years of marriage do, one imagines, have some connection with the expectations and behaviour of the families and guests on the occasion of the reception. I've been to some that were an exercise in a cold and paralysing restraint and others that deteriorated into bawdiness and throwing up behind sofas. Perhaps the central characters went on to be happy ever after but it would be surprising were it totally forgotten by one had the other's guests behaved as if they were at home in their natural pig-sty.

Ella remained at the table sedate and probably nervous. My father's easy affable ways clearly set the example, impressing everyone not least Mrs Burley who batted her eyelashes at him and caused Ella to say 'Mum!' My mother as I expected was ultra-polite and using her trick of saying 'Indeed' as an answer to any remark. Question mark or exclamation mark were optional.

For example:

'The service is very good.'

'Indeed!?'

Thus instilling a slight doubt.

Particularly impressive was my brother Chris's inadvertent impersonation of Marlon Brando in *On the Waterfront.* Though regrettably he didn't say 'I coulda been a contender' the younger guests were re-assured enough by his example to switch with him to beer. The two rogue characters, Ella's sister Betty and my brother Geoff, chose, for once, as far as one could tell, not to cause any disharmony.

Needless to say there was, if not one of our familiar coincidences, certainly a singular moment, when I finally started my entrée, the others having finished dessert. I looked up and the man sitting opposite to me, also starting his meal, was the world's outstanding goalkeeper. The presence of Gordon Banks, who three years or so later was instrumental in winning the 1966 World Cup for England, was a surprise but presumably he was one of the bride's family's guests. We exchanged some chit-chat on football until it dawned on us both that he was on the wrong table and sadly he left to join his Leicester City team-mates elsewhere in the hotel.

Perhaps it was all too overwhelming for me, for it seemed to end very rapidly and ahead of us lay our carefully-planned honeymoon. All our preparation fell in a heap about three o'clock that afternoon when it became apparent that the heavy snow was not lessening and the radio reported roads closed through most of the country. We abandoned our plan of driving to London and drove instead through a swirling snow-storm to our apartment in Grimsby. It was, had we known it, the start of the coldest, most snow-bound winter and spring of the twentieth century. Our anticipated week in London never eventuated. We had intended to visit the capital's famous exhibitions and palaces, the Royal Portrait Gallery, the Victoria and Albert Museum, London Zoo, Hampton Court and others I forget now. We had tickets to several evening theatre performances, notably *My Fair Lady*. Ella had in advance cast herself as Eliza Doolittle and me as an unlikely Professor Higgins and was practising singing:

Just you wait, 'enry 'iggins, just you wait,
You'll be sorry but your tears 'll be too late.

The Natural History Museum was on our list, being not only my favourite London destination but the scene of an unlikely incident about a year earlier when I'd parked my car outside the museum, spent several hours looking at the exhibits and emerged actually to witness my car being driven away by some young hoodlum. I could hardly believe my eyes, but the police excelled themselves by retrieving it within half an hour. Again I'd got lucky. It never occurred to me that luck might not be an inexhaustible reservoir.

X

There is an apparent freedom, I suppose, in a young man or young woman being unmarried but it doesn't bear much examination. Certainly one has no commitment to consider one's wife and possibly children but there are landladies. Several of these spring to mind: two were tyrannical, two kindly and one indifferent, but they all gave one's life another restrictive dimension. With one, for instance, my room, and of course one only ever had one, was so cold that for several months a glass of water at the bedside regularly froze solid. Most of them, reasonably enough, imposed a curfew and none trusted me with a house key. They soon made it clear that knocking at the door at 2am was frowned upon.

With one such lady this happened three times in almost as many nights and produced a furious harangue that left me apologising obsequiously. Circumstances we won't bother with found me outside the door a fourth time. I had always liked Falstaff's remark 'We have heard the chimes at midnight, Master Shallow' but it was much later than that. The only answer was to climb in. My window was open so it should be possible but would involve scrambling onto the garage roof, then up a drainpipe, eventually hauling myself over the window-sill, all this in a freezing drizzle. As my head and shoulders were almost in there were frenzied shouts inside and someone, it was so dark I have no idea who, pushed me back and I slipped and fell onto the garage top. In a confusion of embarrassment and wondering if this was all life had to offer I fled the scene and spent the night in the waiting-room of Sunbury-on-Thames railway station. Experience had taught me that such places were always available, as the great cathedrals used to be, as a sanctuary for the desperate. What irked me most was having left my shoes on the roof, it being easier to climb in stocking feet. The whole thing resembled a parody of Lucky Jim rather than a hapless imitation.

Ella soon introduced common sense into our household and I was thankful for it. Marriage wasn't giving up on freedom, it was in my case giving up on anarchy. The snow continued to fall and People's Park, seen from our front window, became visually more and more like its Russian equivalent. The absence of any traffic made for a pristine silence and in our isolation we might as well have been in a well-furnished igloo. It was, as Ella in her practicality demonstrated, an ideal setting for a honeymoon. She claimed she had years of leeway to catch up.

She did, as I mentioned before, occasionally make a risqué comment but for our ears only. One of her traits when in bed was to push across with her hip and shoulder until on not a few occasions I was so near to falling out that I went round the other side to escape the pressure. When asked to refrain she would say she wanted to be warmed up and dissolve into giggling, adding that that was all men were good for. She did make a minimal concession that they were also good for carrying things. Years later our daughter confirmed this view adding her own husband's minor contribution, that of unscrewing bottle tops.

Never was there the slightest crudity or coarseness in her speech nor had she the flattened, slightly guttural speech of Walnut Place and for that matter most of Lincolnshire. My Cambridge friends claimed to detect this diction in me and would even mirthfully say, 'Coom oop, boottercoop,' which was vexing of them. Ella's articulation was that of her mother, the speech of her home town of Bath, England's most upmarket city where Jane Austen lived for five years, set two of her novels and where ladies and gentlemen assembled to take the waters.

Her idiosyncrasies, Ella's not Jane's, soon expressed themselves. On our first night in our new apartment she disappeared into the bathroom. Thereafter there was only the soft thumps of snow sliding off the roof until I had to ask: 'Are you all right?' She emerged to explain, as to an idiot savant, that a normal bath was a luxury to someone used to huddling in a tub in the kitchen, something which in my hedonism I could hardly be expected to appreciate. Throughout our marriage she was inclined to assume that since every small function, such as filling the bath, had been done for me by my nanny, she, Ella, would have to replace this lady. 'Here take this aspirin – put it in your mouth – take a sip of water and swallow.' Having rarely taken pills I would choke and there would be more chiding: 'Swallow! Don't be a baby.' Pointing out my inexperience with aspirins only prompted her to assume that my nanny had swallowed them for me, followed by accounts of how her own family in times of famine had been reduced to eating used tea-leaves, presumably while my nanny and I were gorging ourselves on pate de foie gras.

What did it matter what she said? I loved and adored her and wanted nothing more than her presence. She has gone now and my world seems very empty.

What of soul was left, I wonder,
when the kissing had to stop?

1963 was a blissful year. One can understand how Wordsworth felt writing:

Bliss it was in that dawn to be alive
But to be young was very heaven.

He was inspired by the thought that the French Revolution's coming was to make life better for millions, but I doubt our simpler happiness was any less than his.

Of course pre-eminently there was Ella's pregnancy in which she rejoiced, soon locating a pre-natal centre and starting activities such as swimming. One eventuality neither of us had foreseen was her craving for various foods. This began with chocolate, more particularly her home-made cakes, large and oozing with chocolate which we both devoured. This appetite changed marginally into her demanding chocolate ices. Usually about 3am she would implore me to go out into the blizzard and bring some back. It seemed, in mid-winter, about as hopeless a quest as hunting down the elixir of everlasting life was for the medieval alchemists, but I tried. In a sense it was the same quest if it helped the life inside her. The choc-ices had to be found. Despite hours of frustration I found them at daybreak and, behold, it was at Wonderland itself at an unpromising kiosk. My first purchase was accompanied by a deluge of icy spray as a large wave swept through the beach-front railings.

'Bit cold for ice-cream, mate,' said a witty newspaper man.

'Not if it guarantees immortality.'

''Ere, I'll 'ave one then.'

Some women, she told me, preferred chalk or soap. My education was diversifying.

Soon after there followed a series of events and a discovery that made me even prouder of her, if that was possible. The snow and ice held Britain in their grip through January, February and even March. Deprived of their football matches the population seemed to be suffering withdrawal symptoms so that when April came the sporting activity was frantic. The head coach of England's Under-21 football team lived in Grimsby and recruited me as an assistant coach. Working at that level was fascinating and the team was due to play West Germany at Wembley

Stadium. Ella made little of my rise to fame for reasons that were shortly to emerge. There came a formal invitation for us to have dinner with the Duke of Edinburgh on the evening before the match. Needless to say this was not a tête-a-tête as there were about forty other guests. Ella protested that she was too tubby but was easily persuaded to disregard this. At the dinner she was lively and bouncy and delighted to find not only that she had a seat next day in the Royal Box at Wembley but that lunch before the game would be in the Queen's Dining Room just behind the box. Sadly, as Ella was a convinced royalist, Her Majesty was elsewhere. The wife of another coach told me the Duke had flirted outrageously with Ella, calling her a bonny lass. She denied this but smiled.

As we drove home she astonished me, almost causing an accident. Quite casually, never having mentioned it before, she remarked that she was familiar with Wembley Stadium, having played hockey there for England. The match had also been against West

Germany, the result exactly the same, a 1–2 loss.

'England!' I gasped astonished. 'At Wembley!'

Why had she never told me? In reverse I would have forced her to listen repeatedly to every minute detail.

'What do you remember of it?'

'The crowd and the noise.' There had been 80,000 people there.

'What else?'

'The German girls! So big, like Amazons.'

'Were you chosen again?'

'Yes, against Wales, but it was a Wednesday and they wouldn't give me time off work.'

She couldn't get a couple of days off work to play for her country? It was a national disgrace! She smiled and said that it didn't matter. She was amazing and so modest. Amazing grace.

Later she produced a newspaper cutting. She earned one sentence but it was enough. It shone out: 'No-one fought harder in the mid-field than Ella Burley'.

'My mother washed my England shirt every day for weeks and kept hanging it out to dry because she wanted everyone to see it.' Of course, well done, Mrs Burley! The little story of the shirt I will never forget because she told me it again the day before she died. Maybe she was thinking of wresting the ball from the Amazons nearly sixty years ago.

'It was white with a red rose.' Too often the words fade but those never will. Never. I can picture her walking out of the dark tunnel into the stadium's light and clamour, running onto the green grass with her red rose.

What a change Ella made in our finances! And why not? It might have been, but for our chance meeting, that the Exchequer would have recruited her. Our finances, in comparison, were child's play. Remarking only that she had not realised she was marrying a bankrupt her account absorbed my deficit and without any exaggeration no financial information came my way until the next century. The debt revealed the cost of her wedding ring which simultaneously pleased and horrified her. The ultimate outrage was mine when one of the demon's lackeys dragged the ring off her finger in the last month of her life and kept it. Can you imagine the scum we share the world with! This particular odious sub-human had left a clue or two and for days I searched the suburbs of Adelaide on its trail, but sadly in vain.

How far into the future that all was! The baby was nearly due and she entered hospital cheerful and confident. It was almost a disaster. Late on the night of Thursday 27th of June she went into labour and the agony that only women know. The baby was misaligned in the womb. I never knew the technicalities. The night passed and all the next day with pain, struggle and no relief. I was full of foreboding as her face was ashen and lined. There seemed to be an apathy or misplaced optimism in the nursing staff. The obvious answer was a caesarean birth but my medical knowledge was so slender I didn't say, 'Get on with it, or I'll sue you for murder'. In the early hours of Saturday the baby was delivered by caesarean section. To my utter relief she was sitting up in bed, her baby at her breast, the pain and fears over.

So she came home triumphant and her mother was there to meet her and insisted on marching around the house carrying the baby, having herself borne six. Mrs B had brought a splendid pram, a pageant in itself, green, almost a barouche with on the side an enamelled plaque of a red rose, her own device. For names we chose Christopher, for my brother's courage and common sense, also Edward for my uncle's manual skills and love of the countryside and Thomas, my grandfather, for honour. The next was to be Ella's choice and she had ready David Henry, but there was to be only one boy.

Needless to say she was the perfect mother. Of course the baby was her constant companion. Among a multitude of hazy impressions three have some clarity. With the grand pram mother and son would parade around People's Park and others out walking would stop and very properly admire such an admirable little boy. Another of his mother's tactics was to allow him to rest in the pram under a large tree so that, as she said, he would look upwards and get acquainted with the natural world and its beauty. Then there were the mandatory visits to relations and their required esteem. The relationship between my mother and Ella began gradually to thaw as a consequence of the baby being declared beautiful, pleasing my wife, and his also being declared closely to resemble the Roe clan, thus gratifying my mother.

Soon came the examinations at Clee, as the school was invariably called. 5A took it seriously and passed everything with airy ease even without having Subversive Rhetoric as an examination subject. Several of them we invited around one evening and excellent company they were, not least because Ella was so at ease with them. This trait never varied throughout my teaching career and Mrs Roe became a friend and confidante of hundreds of boys.

About this time I became a qualified teacher with a licence. My having taught for several years and driven cars for even more years without in either case the cachet of approval by officialdom was now at an end. An accredited teacher and the owner of a driving licence there was little of the maverick left. Goodbye, rebel without a cause. I had little faith in my brand new Diploma of Education. Though quite interesting on the history of education in Britain, it only waffled around the central factor at least as I had grasped and experienced it. This was the modus vivendi between pupils and teacher. It is an aspiration that one approaches or recedes from and rarely does it crystallise into reality. My own conception of it would be too complex to fit into this story but a parallel might be the art of juggling. The juggler keeps his glass balls in the air, two at a time, then three, then more and we wonder at his skill and control for all the balls share equally his energy and attention. Lucky juggler! No juggler has up to thirty balls none of which is alike. In the simplest terms that is the teachers' art. My own History master, a great teacher, described this art as a three-way conversation between himself, the members of the class and the material they were studying. So you and I and Geoffrey Chaucer or perhaps William Pitt the Elder would become engaged in a civilised interaction. My opinion of the Diploma was not unlike Hitler's 'scrap of paper' view of the Munich settlement. Completely different was my decision to take another degree, this time with London University, which I began in mid-1963 and of which more later.

The world of might-have-been is an intriguing one. It is the future one doesn't get to have and presumably some reaction of thankfulness or disappointment that it hasn't eventuated. Only in the parallel universes does one take the other options. Our future took a significant step when our son was only six months old. For this the responsibility was entirely mine. The undertaking was reasonable enough one minute but capricious and chancy the next. It also involved changing the lives of at least two other people, Ella and Christopher.

I came across an advertisement for a teaching position in Rhodesia. Its conditions sounded attractive and it had all the feel of a probable might-have-been, yet also something my sub-conscious had been watching out for, a sort of wild surmise.

> *Then felt I like some watcher of the skies*
> *When a new planet swims into his ken;*
> *Or like stout Cortez when with eagle eyes*
> *He star'd at the Pacific – and all his men*
> *Looked at each other with wild surmise –*
> *Silent – upon a peak in Darien.*

The poetry had a special appeal to me for various reasons: firstly it was Vasco Balboa, not stout Cortez, who was the first European to see the Pacific, and secondly one of my classes at Clee had parodied the final line as 'Silent – upon a peke in Darien'. I don't know if the trope was original but the image reduced me to helpless laughter, though slightly sympathising with the peke and wishing that Cortez's men had stood silently upon my sister's lurcher.

XI

The headmaster of Peterhouse, the Rhodesian school in question, met us for lunch at Lyon's Corner House on Oxford Street, an oddly unfashionable choice. He was charismatic and outspoken and shortly after relating how he had translated Herodotus while camped on the South Col of Everest, then bribing the accordionist to stop playing, he offered us the position. Ella impressed by his bonhomie and his addressing her as 'young lady' felt reassured that this would not be a trip with Joseph Conrad to some hell-hole in the Congo. In retrospect she took the day and the three years that followed so remarkably well that I was proud of her. But then I invariably was.

We left our smart apartment in Grimsby on November 22nd 1963. People tend to remember what they were doing then, the day John F. Kennedy was assassinated. Our flight left on December 31st which gave a month or so for families to commiserate with Ella and Christopher. 'Is the child inoculated against leprosy?' Was my hare-brained irresponsibility the behaviour of a sensible married man I and everyone else wondered. Why do it when one could be eating cod and chips out of a newspaper in the alternative universe of Wonderland!

So we found ourselves in the Southern Hemisphere with the sun disorienting us by shining from the north. In fact most things disoriented us at first. Everything started deceptively well when we spent the first day and night as guests of Mr and Mrs Snell. Their house was smart and airy, its garden glorious and when we walked through the school we were certainly impressed. It was only nine years old but had an imposing chapel and was in many ways akin to British independent schools, at least in its rural setting. It had about three hundred and fifty boys, all boarders.

On day two, the boys being still on holiday, we were shown our house. There were various houses dotted around the property for the staff and their families, all of them pleasant enough places. Ours was very different.

It consisted of two rondavels, circular brick rooms with conical thatched roofs though no ceilings and a third room-cum-passage which joined them. Our furniture had yet to arrive so we had been provided with a bed, a cot, some miscellaneous chairs and so on. Ella, hearing from our nearest neighbour that snakes were frequently found in the thatch of the roofs of the house we had been allocated, remarked in tired exasperation: 'Toto, I've a feeling we're not in Kansas any more.' For some years she had belonged to a film club and was word-perfect in films like *Singing in the Rain* and *South Pacific* and easily capable of quoting from the *Wizard of Oz.*

There was a garden. One look at it and I recognised it at once: 'a large garden, only half-cultivated with bushes as big as summerhouses of Marshal Neil roses, lime and orange trees, clumps of bamboos and thickets of high grass.' Of course! It was the familiar garden of Rikki-tikki-tavi the mongoose. In Kipling's story the man and wife who own the garden have, as did we, one small boy and in the garden live Nag and Nagaina the fearsome cobras, both of whom also appear in the poem *The Female of the Species*. It was our garden for about a week and it had cobras and mongooses all right and it wasn't Grimsby, Toto.

A note to young teachers: if you've an unruly or bored class and you wish to hold them in mesmerised attention read them the tale of Rikki-tikki-tavi. Only *The Man who would be King* can beat it as a story and it's a bit too long to fit into a lesson.

'You can go and see the Head and tell him that we need a proper house,' said Ella, having spent the night with the light on looking up at the interior thatch and listening to anonymous scrapes and rustlings. 'If you don't I will'.

This ultimatum was clearly not open even to the least question but was postponed by a surprise development. Our rondavels were outlying, relative to the rest of the school's buildings, but close to the African village. The village was part of the school's estate and had a population that either grew maize, invariably known as mealies, the staple food of southern Africa, or were employed in a variety of roles by the school. None of this we knew that day, our third in the country, but we started to find out when Lucia arrived. She was a Shona girl, about twenty, tall, good-looking and athletic. She walked up to Ella and announced: 'I have come to work for you.'

'Doing what?' said my wife, thankfully diverted from leaving for England, home and beauty.

'Looking after the baby.'

'I can look after my own baby.'

'First I shall do the washing.' Despite protests Lucia filled a tub with water and washed whatever clothes she could find, beating them with a stone. Then ignoring objections she strewed the clothes out over the thorn bushes in the garden. There were nearly tears at the spectacle.

'The baby is crying,' said Lucia. 'I shall take him for a walk.' Christopher was wrapped in a head-scarf used as a sort of sling, hauled across Lucia's back and they went off together. He had at once stopped crying.

There seemed nothing left to do except point out to Mr Snell that our accommodation, though interesting, was basically a shanty. A stroke of luck came our way in that a member of staff was suddenly appointed to a headship elsewhere. His house when we saw it was deemed satisfactory by both Ella and Lucia. The ball had spun red for the first time in Africa. There remained the problem of Lucia, who seemingly assumed that we now employed her.

Though we had not the slightest idea that this was so, there was a deal of politico-social manoeuvring taking place where Lucia was concerned. Not only had she ignored Ella's fairly natural wish to take care of her own child but had returned next day with a cook, whom she assumed would be at once employed, and told us that she was also looking around for a capable gardener. Ella sacked Lucia, did not appoint Chirra the cook, and said, with little evidence, that I was a capable gardener. Lucia departed, bribed by a large slice of bread and jam, but with a look that said this wasn't the end of it.

The next day Mr Snell requested the pleasure of our company and after some introductory pleasantries asked why we refused to employ the minimum entourage. Ella launched into a justification of her position which essentially was that she felt ill at ease managing servants. Though at first low-key her position became steadily more revolutionary and close to quoting: 'Men are born free and remain equal in rights'. Perhaps it was just as well that particular Jacobinical ruling got side-tracked as the equality of man, and certainly not of women, wasn't Rhodesia's long suit. The Head was unperturbed and asked if our salary was satisfactory. It was, very satisfactory. But jobs for the African villagers were difficult to find. A few pounds, even a few shillings, mean a great deal to some households, Mrs Roe. But of course, my dear, you are perfectly entitled to spend your money as you choose. That is your privilege. Lucia, Chirra and Crispin, our thirteen-year-old gardener, were reinstated the next day and for three years were nominally servants but in fact close friends.

Crispin refused to accept a wage on condition that he could read my books. He would and did go far.

So much for Mr Snell's manoeuvres but there were other politics at work too. Within hours of Ella's arrival at Peterhouse disturbing news swept through the African village, brought home by the school's African employees. A witch had arrived and taken up residence: a bona fide, gun witch, partly recognisable by her arrogant treatment of her husband, which no African woman could conceive of, but much more so by her long red hair. African witches always had red hair, but dyed with clay and therefore not quite the genuine article. The new power-house witch must be kept on side, which is why Lucia, only daughter of the village chieftain Ezekiel, was chosen to conduct a reconnaissance.

The duo of Ella and Lucia fizzed and sparkled like the very air of this new country. Perhaps it was a side-effect of living at five thousand feet as all of central Rhodesia was on a high plateau. Perhaps it was the scents of wood-smoke and msasa trees. These were shapely trees, millions of them, their young leaves a memorable amber-purple, stretching away on all sides in this beautiful almost empty land. Life felt like an adventure in a way that Britain could never provide. But we knew that Britain was our homeland and sanctuary and just as well when the adventure showed signs of turning into an ordeal.

The school, Peterhouse, was an admirable institution. Its remoteness gave it a self-assurance and unity. The staff was highly-qualified and committed with a strong contingent from Oxford's Oriel College drawn by the Head, himself an Oriel man. A number of the staff had had other professions and backgrounds unlike almost all my colleagues in English schools. There was a blend of different nationalities with a number of expatriate British.

The curriculum and examination system were little different from that at Clee, indeed the Cambridge Certificate of Education was exactly the same. The chief difference lay in the boys themselves. They were high-spirited, independent and ready to learn. There was nothing of the English trade union approach of a block of pupils, sometimes as many as half of a class, prepared to do just enough to remain comfortably anonymous spectators. Or maybe I had not been sufficiently stimulating. I'm not sure. Perhaps I'm being unfair. Many of the Rhodesian boys were of farming stock and used to the wild isolated lives of the cattle and tobacco farms. They were natural sportsmen, loving cricket and rugby, and in 1989 actually won the World Schools' Rugby competition.

Ella integrated at once into the dual societies of staff and boys. She would regularly call for aid to remove snakes from the garden and would reward the boys with home-made lemonade. The Great Snake War became a priority when one day she put Christopher outside in the garden in his pram protected by mosquito netting, then only minutes later found a snake reclining on the net as if in a hammock. She hurled it away with laundry tongs only, as I heard later, to be admonished by the boys she summoned to help: 'Mrs Roe, how can you be so unkind!' The snake was then comforted and placed in a walled pit owned by the large and dedicated Herpetological Society. On one occasion the herpetologists took Christopher into the pit so that he could 'see better'. Ella put her foot down and for several months upset the boys by referring to the snakes as 'serpents'.

A memorable moment occurred when my analysis of whether *The Tempest* was a comedy, a tragedy, or neither, was diverted by a snake's head emerging from Pete Webber's shirt pocket.

'Webber, is that a real snake, or is this an alternative universe?'

'Sir, it is a pet.' Obviously, said his tone and demeanour. Like a harmless bunny rabbit.

'And if it bit you?'

'That would be a comedy' said the others.

'And if it bit your classmates?'

'That would be a tragedy,' they said, not unreasonably.

'And if it bit me?'

'That would be neither. It would be like the storm in *The Tempest*. An act of God.'

And what's more they were right. They must have been paying attention.

In February Ella announced that she was pregnant. Not to be outdone Lucia also announced her pregnancy, though not yet having acquired a husband. We acquired a dog. This was no ordinary dog. At first he was just an unco-ordinated bundle of over-sized paws and ears. He was an Alsatian and we called him Nimrod, the great grandson of Noah and 'a mighty hunter' according to Genesis. In what seemed no time Nimrod became huge, by far the most powerful German Shepherd (to use his other title) I've ever seen. He was handsome and intelligent with a thick creamy ruff and feared nothing. Ella loved and indulged him and called him Nimmy. Lucia was less than impressed, particularly when taking Chris out in his pram she had to be accompanied by Nimrod. I can hear her now: 'Madam, not Neemee, don't let Neemee come.' Lucia knew perfectly well that Nimrod would not allow any of Lucia's many suitors anywhere near the pram and she would have only the boring company of other nannies.

Ella liked to take Chris swimming, or at least for a dip in the school pool, and would be at her wits' end with Nimrod who would jump in and shepherd mother and child to the steps thus saving their lives. Lucia puzzled over this and clearly disapproved of my wife's complaisancy. Nimrod deserved to be given a strong dose of the occult and who better to administer it than madam.

Marandellas was a small town about five miles away and the area's only real settlement in wide sweeps of bushland. Ella shopped there from time to time, often accompanied by Nimrod who could not bear being away from her for long. On such occasions he stayed inside the car, being far too powerful and self-willed to be constrained by a lead. On one occasion he got out of the car and blithely accompanied Ella to the open-air market. Here he encountered Simba, an equally huge black Alsatian, and the fight was a source of conversation for years. Apparently the combatants were obscured for much of the time by an almost biblical pillar of dust and my wife, to her credit, went into this cloud to separate them. It was, of course, hopeless and a question of waiting to see who won. Nimrod was victorious and we were besieged with offers to buy him, offers which reached half a year's worth of my salary. We have never had, or wanted, another dog since.

From being very young Ella had spent much time next door at 4 Walnut Place with her grandmother. From her she had learned the skill of sewing and had become adept at the mysterious art of needlework. Even its vocabulary was arcane. What were needlepoint, crochet, cross-stitch, appliqué to name only a few, to say nothing of lace, an artifice all of its own? She was at the time only moderately interested in dressmaking which did not prevent the headmaster's wife, personally supervising the staff families' decorum, remarking to me: 'It is deplorable that there are only two stylishly-dressed women in this whole place. One is your wife, the other is that nanny of hers.'

Speech Day arrived so Ella made herself an elegant hat. She liked social occasions, though in my experience

Speech Days had the same soporific effect as eating too much lettuce had, according to Beatrix Potter, on Peter Rabbit. But this was not so with Peterhouse's headmaster. Knowing his speech would appear in the press he launched into a fiery political attack on the government's racial policy. He was right to do so and right to offer scholarships to African pupils. The heart of the problem was obvious enough: the political system enabled white Rhodesians, a minority of at most one twentieth of the population, to form the government. Short of a decision to grasp the nettle and enfranchise the coloured Rhodesians the future was likely to be, and was, tragic. The numbers simply wouldn't add up. Had enfranchisement been enacted fairly and generously the history of the country might have been very different. As it turned out the next few decades were to bring massacre, misery, famine and social and economic disintegration into a pariah state under the dictatorship of a Marxist psychopath. Marxist economics being what they are it is unsurprising that Zimbabwe, as Rhodesia is now called, has a Stone Age economy with a currency so worthless that in 2015 an egg cost 50 billion Zimbabwean dollars and they were printing 100 trillion dollar notes.

However, back to October 1964, a sad month for us. One Saturday found me in Salisbury, the country's stylish and attractive capital city, coaching the School's cricket team. A phone call reached me to say that Ella was being rushed to the city's major hospital, several days earlier than we had anticipated, and the baby was due that afternoon. Then things cascaded out of control. The baby was born either dead or dying shortly after birth, I cannot say. I never found out. Other than this we never kept secrets from one another. It was a girl, which Ella had hoped for and she had even chosen a name, Charlotte. When the wheel spun it was an unfortunate truth that sometimes you weren't sure what exactly the stakes were. There were we betting that this time it would be a girl and it was and it was not. No doubt the demon would have thought that a clever little conceit.

'Nothing is but what is not,' said Macbeth in despair as he sank further into the cruel world of might-have-been. 'What might little Charlotte have been?' Ella once asked me.

'Someone special,' I said. Probably I should have said nothing. I don't know.

Though it would have been sensible to stay in hospital she refused to do so and consequently we drove back to Peterhouse, about fifty miles, in a truck. The school had several of these trucks and often used them to transport sporting teams, the master-in-charge or the coach driving. The night was moonless and wet, the cab was cold and the road rutted and pot-holed. She never spoke, though I tried a few times to converse, until we reached our house. 'A nice way to come home,' she said. I don't like writing about it and try not to think back to that black night and the rain sliding and sidling across the windscreen. It was nearly the worst day of my life, though there would be plenty of days in the future vying to be a thorn in that crown.

Though no-one would have denied her a period of mourning, this was given a different perspective by a telegram from my mother announcing that she would be shortly arriving at Salisbury airport. She came with her usual challenging flourish, perhaps drawn from the Victorian music-hall song:

No! No!! No!!! When we go to meet the foe
It's the English-speaking race against the world.

In no time the cool relationship between the two ladies began to warm. My mother had not lost a baby but had lost her two sisters, both dying of diabetes as teenagers. Her remedy for Ella's sadness was to organise an adventurous trip around the country lasting several weeks. 'We'll work it out as we go,' she said, probably expecting to use her expertise in booking rooms in Vienna's fashionable hotels. We drove south to Bulawayo and then to the granite and kopjes of the Matopos hills where we stood at the grave of Cecil Rhodes. Huge multi-coloured lizards wandered around our feet and the rolling boulder-strewn landscape seemed as empty and lonely as if we had somehow found ourselves on the planet a million years ago.

On we drove, around us the msasas stretching to the horizon. Without even entering a reservation we had twenty elephants tramping past our stationary car. Ella cried out, 'Oh, look at the babies,' and we hoped she saw only the small elephants. Wherever we went there were giraffes, the most graceful of animals. For a quarter of an hour a buffalo barred the road in front of us. A huge crocodile emerged from a waterhole nearby. Everywhere we saw antelopes, wildebeestes and zebras. In later years a film called *Jurassic Park* had the same sense of wonder at the prehistoric creatures. That was before the part where various people were dismembered by velociraptors. The film was nothing new to someone like me brought up on Conan Doyle's *The Lost World;* as a boy in Upper Third my ambition was to be either Clive of India or Lord John Roxton, hero of Doyle's novel. I was well at home in a fictional jungle. Ella who at thirteen saw herself as an emerging jazz singer had several times been to Ella Fitzgerald concerts. I had to admit her ideal was the more realistic. But that's a diversion.

On we went to Victoria Falls. It is sublimely spectacular. Is there any wonder on Earth that can compare with The Smoke that Thunders? We were transfixed and she and I made a pact to come back again one day. I took a boat-trip on the Zambezi, leaving Ella to feed Christopher on an island in the river. 'Perfectly safe', said our guide. We returned from the hippos and crocs to find a monkey had stolen Christopher's milk bottle and biscuits and frayed Ella's patience, so much so that the monkey was whacked with a stick.

We followed the Zambezi eastwards until we reached the enormous Kariba Dam, not quite finished but a mighty construction and already Lake Kariba was forming behind it, changing the world's atlases. We sat that night on our hotel verandah watching the monsoon break with a display of pyrotechnics beyond belief. Was Ella forgetting Charlotte? I didn't know. I suppose not.

Before we set out for Rhodesia I had decided to take another degree, this time in English. At least my lessons would have some legitimacy. There would be little or no access to tuition or libraries or even adequate book shops which made it all a daunting prospect. With this in mind I had, while still in England, studied the past papers of the examination. There were nine papers: six were based on periods of English Literature, one was entirely on Shakespeare, the other two were Anglo-Saxon and Philology. I never did grasp Philology, which really required tuition, so I needed to pass the rest. The literary papers each required three essays in three hours, so the answer seemed to be to choose three major authors from each period and pray there was a question on each of them. It meant being proficient in eighteen major authors. Shakespeare I liked anyway and could even teach him with snakes in the audience.

It sounded possible and interesting. But I couldn't afford two failures, so what was to be done about Anglo-Saxon. 'I'm not confident about Anglo-Saxon,' I told Ella. One of her automatic assumptions was that a simple everyday task, e.g. ironing a handkerchief, would baffle me but some lofty and scholarly enterprise would be child's play.

'Well, learn it,' she said. 'I'll help you.'

This we set out to do. It was fascinating. Gradually the strange language made sense, as if a thousand years had faded away. One had to accept its idiosyncrasies: four of its letters we no longer use and five of ours didn't exist then or were very rare. Also it was a declension language which always complicates things, other than to Latin adepts like Ella, who claimed learning Latin was 'fun and easy'. After a while things became less like decoding the Rosetta Stone and more like an absorbing game. My wife with her Aslackoe and wapentake connections liked the sound of the language and sometimes would ask me to go into the next room and recite Anglo-Saxon poetry. She said that, muffled by the door, it sounded like the past talking to her. She particularly liked the Lord's Prayer:

Faeder ure thu the eart on heofonum
Si thin nama gehalgod
To becume thin rice
Gewurthe thin willa
On eorthan swa swa on heofonum

All the 'th' sounds used to be letters we no longer have, otherwise this is the language of about 1000AD. I liked the word 'rice' (pronounced rick) meaning kingdom. One finds it still in, for instance, 'bishopric' or indeed the German 'reich'.

Some things were favourable. There was no television and, being in the tropics, night came early. But no advantage came close to Ella's breadth of intellect, no reinforcement close to her encouragement. In the papers on the major authors it seemed to me that while I provided the commentary, as it were, the authors should speak for themselves. Assume no idea, interpret nothing, until you've appraised and quoted their actual words. It meant learning literally thousands of lines and you can guess who patiently rehearsed me through them.

She was smart and perceptive and inclined to pour cold water on abstruse literary criticism, sometimes calling it 'psycho-babble' in her mathematical desire for clarity. One such example came from the play *Macbeth*. The actions and thoughts of Macbeth and Lady Macbeth have produced enough critical texts of one sort or another to stretch from Scotland to the moon. 'No,' said Ella. 'They do what they do, they think what they think, because they love one another, no more and no less.'

'Surely the witches changed his thinking,' I suggested.

'Charlatans! Forget them and all that stuff about boiled toads.' I don't read or watch the play any more. They loved one another to distraction (and destruction) but Lady Macbeth developed Alzheimer's. Read the text and tell me if I'm wrong. For a start listen to this:

Macbeth: 'How does your patient, doctor?'

Doctor: 'Not so sick, my lord, as she is troubled with thick-coming fancies
That keep her from her rest.
Macbeth: 'Cure her of that.
Canst thou not minister to a mind diseased,
Pluck from the memory a rooted sorrow,
Raze out the written troubles of the brain...?'

Shakespeare never knew the term 'Alzheimer's' but he knew the symptoms all right, and if what happened isn't a tragedy I don't know what is.

The whole project of the external degree was demanding but stimulating and among my happier decisions. One feature of the studies involved surprised me at first (though it shouldn't have) and that was how the two disciplines, History and English, refined and defined one another. Toussaint l'Ouverture after leading the slave revolt that led to Haiti's independence was dying in one of Napoleon's prisons when Wordsworth wrote of him:

*Thy friends are exaltations,
agonies,
And love, and man's unconquerable
mind.*

Toussaint's story is moving enough without the poetry but that final line gives it, as literature should, a universality when event or account is transformed into an idea.

The examination took place in Marandellas Methodist Chapel. It lasted a whole week. Philology was a disaster and Medieval Literature nearly was but the others compensated and earned a degree I was quite proud of. A month later I was, according to my wife, 'going round all high and mighty' and not without reason having been awarded two London University prizes, one for Shakespeare and the other (thank you, Ella) for Anglo-Saxon.

XII

Life was such fun, technicoloured in fact, vivid and brimful. Ella became pregnant again. This time it all seemed smoother and far easier for her, and for me as I was despatched only to hunt down liquorice. Fortunately the Marandellas general store stocked it. This time our local GP, 'Doc' Jeffers, was in charge. He didn't mess around and quickly delivered the baby in a caesarean birth in the early morning of 21st December 1965. Christopher, Lucia and I drove to the hospital at daylight. Mother and baby were sitting up looking lively and well. The baby had wispy red hair. Several African nurses gathered around Lucia and began an increasingly noisy conference, speaking in Shona. 'What's all that about?' I said to 'Doc' Jeffers who spoke Shona well.

'I've no idea,' he said. 'Something about a baby witch.'

His remark carried to Lucia and her new friends who took it as medical confirmation of their suspicions, though the baby's red hair was surely evidence enough.

A few days later Juliet was introduced into the household. Juliet was about sixteen, small, pretty and, when not overwhelmed by being installed at Hogwarts, was a devoted nanny. She could naturally not be anything but a junior nanny since Lucia by this time had had two babies herself, calling the first Ella and the second Christopher. Some time later she had another and mysteriously called him Cassius. I was not expecting a namesake, knowing that I only ranked fourth out of four in our household; though having the courtesy title 'Master' it was a token authority. Ella was once warned by Lucia that for some domestic misdemeanour the 'Master' would beat her.

'That would be very unwise, Lucia.'

'What would you do, madam?'

'Something terrible.'

It must have been convincing as soft-hearted Juliet burst into tears. Some slight prestige came my way thanks to my acquaintance with Ezekiel. On several occasions when we had been out to dinner or to some school event Lucia had acted as babysitter and afterwards I had walked with her back to the African village. After several such visits Ezekiel suggested staying and having a beer. Looking back it all seems an illusion. More often than not I had been to some black-tie affair but regardless we sat on stools leaning against the wattle-and-daub of Ezekiel's hut. Even after midnight nobody seemed to be asleep.

'Get yourself a beer, bhasa,' said Ezekiel, kindly elevating me to the same rank as himself. The beer was in a large help-yourself cauldron and in the flickering firelight it was just possible to make out some lumps floating in the liquid.

'What's the stuff in the beer, Ezekiel?'

'Rats, bhasa.'

'Good-oh.'

Not only *The Lost World* but also *King Solomon's Mines* had been formative books in my childhood. I was used to the harrowing perils that Victorian heroes faced with a grin. It was only rat beer not a Zulu impi. In any case it had more flavour than the dish-water known and served in English pubs as 'mild'. Cheers, Ezekiel.

Ella loved her son and her new and precious daughter and loved being with them while surrounded by nannies, cook, gardener, Nimrod and Sammy, an appalling jungle-cat. For most of her life she had owned and was fond of cats, and they, not behaving like their usual selfish selves for once, reciprocated this fondness. Her Australian cats, Lottie and Pete, when not fighting snakes and killing rabbits, were particularly lavish in their affections. Both ignored me other than being resentful if I sat beside her.

She was for once slightly flustered for a week or so while I was away camping with about thirty boys and several of my colleagues. This was because one of the senior boys was so convinced that she was lonely in my absence that he came and sat beside her between about eight and ten o'clock 'in case she was nervous'. She was too kind to terminate this infatuation at once and only did so when presented with a poem dedicated to her charm and aura. In fact the young man concerned, not inaptly named Hugo Folly, was a talented and likable student. At my suggestion that Hugo was missing his mother my wife got quite huffy. She did agree (though perhaps a trifle reluctantly) that staff members' wives should not behave like Delilah.

The expedition with the boys had taken us to the Chimanimani Ranges on the border with Mozambique. It was completely uninhabited, a wild and beautiful plateau which today is one of Africa's finest game reserves. Several boys climbed with me to its highest point and half-way back to our camp-site it occurred to me that my expensive camera was still on the peak. It was hard work reclimbing the mountain particularly when time was lost evading an aggressive troupe of baboons. Fortunately the camera was there. In the twilight I got partly off the mountain but had to find a place to sleep. At dawn I woke in a dense fog to hear feet moving and a sound like cows cropping grass. Five minutes later a gust of wind split the fog and around me was a herd of elands, Africa's giant and gentle antelope, probably thirty of them. I watched for an hour. Maybe the Garden of Eden was like that.

But elsewhere in the country the signs were ominous. Terrorist activity was slight and usually in remote parts or on the country's borders. In 1964 and 1965 it hardly seemed to matter. But in 1966 it began to creep inwards from Zambia, Mozambique and Angola. There were primitive ambushes, even in the friendly country around Marandellas. Twice on lonely dirt roads I drove round a corner to see a pole barring the way. The recommended response was to spin off the road onto the verge, which was usually sparse, crash through the undergrowth and back onto the road beyond the barrier. It worked for me but it was an adrenalin rush. Lucky again.

Ella and Chirra, our cook, also struck lucky, at least in her opinion. She was a very good cook herself though underplaying her skills. My colleagues on the staff invited us to dinner from time to time and when we, or rather she, reciprocated there were forebodings and certain ladies known to be elite cooks were asked out to restaurants instead (or the restaurant, as Marandellas had only one that ventured beyond 'mealie' combinations). Her first major enterprise as 'the hostess with the mostest' met an unexpected and unorthodox end. The entrée came and went conventionally enough, and then was produced boeuf stroganoff for twelve, a dish she had never created before. It looked all right but before anyone managed a mouthful there was a fearful crash of thunder and lightning struck the house. I remember the telephone sprang vertically out of its socket and hit the ceiling and half a dozen light bulbs exploded, decorating the stroganoffs with an incrustation of finely-shattered glass. The dishes were immediately whisked away. 'Thank heaven for that,' she whispered to me in the kitchen. 'It'll save us having our stomachs pumped.'

'Surely we wouldn't have eaten the glass?' I said.

'It wasn't the glass I was worried about.' She never made boeuf stroganoff again. It was deemed unlucky. But there came a spell when things went consistently well for us, despite frequent unpromising situations from which somehow we extricated ourselves.

Luck exists. From a common sense point of view it exists. It's all very well determinists arguing that every infinitesimal event since the world began, every drop of rain that falls, combines to create one unavoidable present and future. Maybe, nor shall we ever know. But it's like the duck: if it looks like luck, behaves like luck and is indistinguishable from luck, then it's luck. Ask the cricket captain spinning the coin. Better still ask the great tragedian Aeschylus who had remarkably ill luck in 456BC when an eagle, believing his head to be a rock, dropped a tortoise on him, killing him. Considering eagles have marvellous eyesight and this eagle was presumably fairly close to Aeschylus that does seem unlucky. My sympathies are with him, not least because he wrote: 'There is no pain so great as the memory of joy in present grief.'

I know, Aeschylus, I know.

Our third and final year in Rhodesia overflowed with potential debacles. The first followed a decision by two of my colleagues and me to set out to climb Kilimanjaro, driving there in a Kombi van. The mountain is in Tanzania, on the border with Kenya, and for us was about 1200 miles away. Our research and preparation were close to non-existent, though we did take our golf clubs in case we should pass attractive golf-courses on the way. Almost all our journey was on dirt roads where the corrugations gave one a sort of St Vitus Dance even when stationary. Among the hazards was crossing the Kwambe River on a ferry made of planks on oil drums, with a bask of crocodiles accompanying us, only just under water, no doubt anticipating the ferry would overturn as it had only a week before. We drove merrily through the Congo unaware that we were in it or that it was the most violent and anarchic place on earth, until we actually exited it.

Then came a moment of sheer terror. Driving after dark in Africa is, or was then, asking for trouble, but we were close to Kilimanjaro and just about to stop when we were hit by a huge articulated lorry, without lights as usual, this being commonplace in most parts of Africa, and driven by a fourteen-year-old boy, again as usual. The Kombi was flung off the road, rolling down a steep bank and rotating three times as it fell. The impact was so violent I can still hardly believe we were not all killed. Amazingly the vehicle could still move once we got it out of the gully into which we'd rolled, provided we jettisoned almost all our stuff (though not the golf clubs) and thereafter drove at about 10mph. We abandoned Kilimanjaro, though it was a breathtaking sight as we passed with its glaciers glittering in the sun. We chugged along past this superb mountain and almost accidentally reached another marvel, the mighty Serengeti plain and the Ngorogoro Crater. It is a huge extinct volcano, the caldera walls 2000 feet high and the crater's interior a hundred square miles. It was and is rich with Africa's iconic animals and today averages 1500 visitors per day. We ventured down into Africa's wonderland and saw only three other people but an endless parade of splendid animals and birds.

Our battered van had so many half-attached pieces of metal that it jangled as it moved, sounding like a primitive xylophone. We reached Mombasa and sold it for what it was, scrap. David left us for the sanity of England and Radley College, rather as if one of Ulysses' sailors had jumped ship, tired of the perils of their wanderings. Without the van Eddie and I were reduced to strolling through the seething streets of Mombasa holding our golf clubs and earning undeserved respect as otherworldly mendicants or mystics.

Anxious to get back but close to penniless we snagged a place on a tramp steamer bringing pilgrims south from Mecca en route to places like Zanzibar or Lourenco Marques. It also stopped at Beira which had a railway link to Rhodesia. We were undeterred by the Mombasa harbour-master warning us that no European had ever been on this trip. We certainly didn't gorge ourselves at the buffet since a day's tucker consisted of a slice of bread and several cups of tea.

I made a phone call from Beira to Peterhouse asking Ella to pick us up at Thaydon Kopje, not far from the school, where on an uphill gradient the train slowed down just enough for us to jump off. She was there (I knew she would be) sitting with Christopher and Nimrod on a rug in the shade of the kopje. She looked very attractive and had more eye-shadow and perfume than one normally meets out in the savannah.

'Have you had anything to eat?' she asked.

'I had a slice of bread yesterday.'

'When we get back home we'll have a nice cup of tea.'

'Bravo,' I said.

As we drove back there was an inquisition: why had I only sent one postcard in seven weeks, when did I last shower and why had I not had a haircut?

'No beauty salons in the Masai country.'

'Any golf courses?' she asked.

Outside our house was a welcoming committee of Lucia, Chirra, Crispin and Juliet, holding tight to Madeleine lest Lucia exert her seniority and demand to carry the baby-witch.

'Now,' said Ella, 'Chirra and Crispin can have the day off. Lucia and Juliet and Nimrod can take the children for a long walk. A long walk, Lucia.'

'Oh, madam,' said Lucia.

'Oh, madam,' said Juliet.

'Yes,' said Ella. 'I'm ready for a nice cup of tea.'

About a week before my love died she asked me whether I remembered the evening I got back from the long safari.

'Ah, yes, I remember it well.'

A dirt road ran alongside our garden but in every other direction the garden faded into unfenced bushland or forest, without any real border or definition. Various wild creatures would pass through. A giant python came down past the verandah and away down the road, as did a hyena. A nastier visit was one that must have occurred in the night. At daylight a sheet of grubby paper on the lawn caught my eye. It told me ungrammatically and in boastful capitals that I and my family were on a death-list. It merely confirmed our decision to return to England at the end of that year, 1966. I only told Ella years later.

Not that she was easily intimidated. One of her favourite anecdotes was of the weekend we spent in a remote cottage aptly called World's View. High on a plateau on the Mozambique border one could look out from it across vast empty distances. She had stayed with Christopher, I having driven off to fetch food, when there was a resounding knock on the door. 'Who is it?' she called. There was another knock. 'Who's there?' A third loud knock; apprehensively she opened the door to find herself eye-to-eye with a large secretary bird, the size of an emu.

'What did you do?' I asked, after being chided for abandoning her.

'I drove it away with a towel.'

'How can you be so unkind, Ella?'

'Easily,' she said.

But her tour de force was still to come. She spent a fair amount of time in the African village and had started two very successful clubs there. One was netball, which she played competently and with gusto, the other was sewing, where she was (or would have been had it been India) a guru. The African ladies had a sort of community room and she kept her own sewing-machine there and taught sewing in return for being taught lace-making. As a witch I thought she was losing a bit of edge, certainly compared with Baba Yaga. The latter was a real humdinger of a witch who terrified children in Eastern Europe and Russia for centuries, unsurprisingly as she flew around forests in a mortar, using a pestle as the rudder, had iron teeth and ate human flesh. Nor was that all. She had a hut which could run on large chicken legs and was as lethal as Baba Yaga herself. A pity she or her hut didn't show up on the occasion I'm about to describe, when my red-haired witch showed her scary side.

It began when I came back from school to find my wife interrogating Lucia. 'Look at this!' she said, showing me Lucia's wrist. It was swollen to twice its normal size and no wonder as a sort of bracelet of about forty inch-long thorns from the infamous Rhodesian cactus, the Crown of Thorns, was forming a three-deep band around her wrist. Already it was turning a deep purple and oozing pus. Ella began to extract a thorn or two but Lucia pulled away.

'No, madam, you must leave them.'

'Leave you to get tetanus or gangrene or something. Not likely!'

'The witch-doctor', protested Lucia, 'will be angry.'

'Did he put them in?'

'Yes, madam, to drive out evil.'

'Nonsense,' said Ella. 'They're coming out.' And so they did. A thick layer of antiseptic was applied. 'Now we're going back to the village.'

'Oh, madam.'

'Don't worry about the juju man, Lucia. I'll deal with him.'

There sounded as if there might be fireworks aplenty so I tagged along, possibly as a supernumerary, possibly not. As we were about to enter the village she took some different shoes out of her bag. They were red with very high heels. In the village square, surrounded by people, though all keeping a respectful distance, was the witch-doctor, a massive figure, stripped to the waist and rolling his eyes.

'If you should even think of putting thorns in my nanny's wrist again,' began Ella, and I thought for an apprehensive moment that she meant to continue, '...my husband will give you a damned good thrashing here and now.' What in fact she did say was, '...and I find you here tomorrow I shall turn you into a toad and then put the heel of my shoe right through you.' She gave a realistic demonstration of this action, even pivoting on her stiletto as it bored through the hypothetical toad. The crowd swayed and whispered. Pity we can't recruit Baba Yaga, I thought. And her hut.

'I'll be back in the morning,' said my wife. 'Don't be here. I'm warning you. And, shame on you, Ezekiel, you should look after your daughter better.'

There was no doubt whatsoever that I found Ella bewitching. Anyone who has read thus far can hardly have missed the common thread of my fascination. I was certainly not going to see her embarrassed by some voodoo trafficker so I rang Edgar Mitchell, Peterhouse's security guard, and explained the situation. Edgar had much in common with Rambo and it was only about sixty-forty that he wouldn't make things worse. But sixty-forty! That's more like it!

'OK,' he said. 'Come by my place tomorrow morning.' Edgar had a flock of free-range turkeys and according to Ella the turkeys normally rushed out in an importunate mob and pecked at her calves. She mistrusted large feathered creatures and would relate old wives tales of swans breaking one's leg with a flap of their wings. In Australia she refused to offer peanuts to harmless emus. This time, however, the turkeys, clearly overawed, preferred to disperse as she waded through them. In the village the crowd parted before us like the waters of the Red Sea and we strode through the rondavels into the space at the village centre.

'Where is he?' said my wife. My heart and my head both told me this was all going to end in tears and that shows how much I knew.

Ezekiel came over to me: 'He's gone, bhasa.'

'Lucky for him,' said Ella.

Lucky for us, I thought. But then somebody's got to win the jackpot.

'Will he come back, Ezekiel?' I asked.

'Lucia is my only child. Madam made me ashamed,' he said. Thank heaven for anti-climaxes, at the right moment of course. Ella and the ladies went off in a gaggle to do some collaborative and celebratory sewing while Edgar, Ezekiel and I had a festive rat-beer. One day it was all going to go wrong. Law of averages. But not that day.

I walked back with Edgar. He was limping slightly.

'You OK, Edgar?'

'Just a bit stiff,' he said and pulled a sawn-off shotgun out of his trouser leg. 'Never thought we'd need it.'

'Didn't you.'

'Not after she told Ezekiel to look after his own daughter.'

The world of coincidences tapped me on the shoulder shortly after the rumble in the jungle between Ella and the medicine-man thankfully failed to eventuate. Once again I found myself driving one of the school's trucks back from Salisbury with the Peterhouse rugby team riding in the back. It was pitch black and not far out of the city the road ran alongside the edge of the biggest African township. There was a crash, the windscreen shattered completely into spiked splinters, and a brick (not a half-brick either) bounced up off the steering wheel and landed in my lap. Somehow I held the vehicle steady, coasted to a stop and got out to inform the boys what had happened. They were not there. No-one at all was there, save obviously me wondering how soon it would be before the mob with machetes showed up. Not stopping the vehicle at all would have been the sensible option. Fortunately the boys themselves showed up a few dark, lonely minutes later, escorting an elderly, very frail, white-haired African gentleman, even wheeling his bike for him.

'Here you are, sir. Found him! He was hiding in the bush!'

'No, boys, no. Don't be stupid!' I gave the old man a cigar that fortuitously I'd found in the truck and was hoping to smoke on the way home. We drove away and thankfully that was that. Occasionally it occurs to me how fortunate I have been to have known the pupils who came my way. These lads had jumped out of the truck and plunged straight into the bush in the dark! Nobody throws bricks at us, nor at sir! No wonder their children won the World Schools' Rugby Cup! I expect they would have disapproved of my one-sided incident with the washed-out private detective, as in retrospect so did I. But the detective had upset Ella, so he'd crossed the line just as another person, an uncouth, swaggering lout, was to do in the near future.

The time came for us to leave Peterhouse and Rhodesia and entrain for the long journey south to Cape Town. The farewells were utterly sad. The country was by now under trade sanctions from much of the so-called civilised world. We couldn't even take our furniture out of the country. Ella went to bid farewell to the African village and collect the sewing machine she had inherited from her grandmother. As she told me later the sad faces of the African ladies, as it was the only machine the sewing-club owned, were too much. If it's still there perhaps they still talk of the red witch, who left it behind. In World War II no country in the allied forces had taken more deaths per capita than the white Rhodesians. So whom did Britain choose to betray? Do you need to ask?

My mother, you may remember, was the organist at St Mark's Church in Lincoln. She had the dubious pleasure of listening, for a while, to a pharisaical sermon by some progressive cleric on the need to betray, then rose from her seat and remarked in a voice that rang from apse to font: 'What do you know about it, you ass!' What happened thereafter remains to me a mystery, other than that St Thomas's Church in Heighington at once gained a new organist and St Mark's lost one.

It was a long slow journey to the Cape, crossing two great deserts, the Kalahari and the Karoo. One of our days on the train was Madeleine's first birthday. Against my earnest advice Ella rushed out onto the platform at some desolate stop in the Karoo. I saw her left on the platform as the train moved on.

'Listen, children,' I tried to say, for they were but infants, 'your mother is stranded in the Karoo but we'll probably meet her again at some point in the future, perhaps when the next train reaches Cape Town.' The children, at once missing her, grew fretful, but the train rattled on. After a considerable time and to my huge surprise and relief she strode into our compartment and launched in to a 'How could you abandon me?' sort of one-sided dialectic, not to be diverted or placated by any reminder that she had been advised against the foolhardiness of leaving the train.

She was holding a bun and a candle to stick on it and celebrate Madeleine's first birthday, the celebration lacking some merriment until we had had a lengthy and vivid description of hurling herself into the guard's van, then walking the full length of the train to reach us, since we inevitably were just behind the locomotive, leaving her some twenty-odd carriages to traverse.

Sooner or later, it seemed to me, my, or our, luck would expire or at best we'd just continue to scrape by in the wearying fashion of Lucky Jim. This was a particularly short-sighted and non-existentialist view. Not that I minded being excluded from the philosophies of Jean Paul Sartre. After all, how could I be a free agent controlling my life through acts of the will when other people were throwing bricks through my windscreen?

Time to describe two very different incidents or predicaments. The first and more trivial came on a golf course. A friend of a friend in Cape Town invited me to partner him against another couple who turned out to be furniture tycoons. The golf was good, less so was losing three and two, and deeply embarrassing was being told that we owed them about three hundred rand each. This was entirely due to my customary response to the usual pre-match rigmarole of what stakes are we playing for and so on: instead of saying 'Play you for a couple of drinks' I left this to my partner who had clearly been misled by my Jay Gatsby persona.

Ella and I had got three hundred rand, just, but we also had to live for a fortnight in Cape Town and several days on the liner home.

I suppose there were sensible options, in fact plenty of them, almost an inexhaustible supply, but our opponents had had the rub of the green so far, at least in my opinion, and in a hare-brained moment I suggested playing double or quits for the cash. A birdie on the 17th and we got ahead. A half on the next, please, and we're home. My partner put me in a dense thorn thicket and I could only hack it out backwards. He hit a flaky sort of three-wood reaching the edge of the green. Our opponents were placidly on the green in two. The only hope was holing this enormous putt. I thought about semi-collapsing and feigning some dreadful condition: 'I should never have played – it's the old asthma you know.' Perhaps it was the thought of the hapless Piggy in *Lord of the Flies* that stopped me. What had Piggy said: 'My aunty told me not to play golf on account of my asthma.' Actually his aunty in the novel had told him 'not to run' but the predicament was the same. Anyway the furniture tycoons could easily have read *Lord of the Flies* and could justifiably quote the response Piggy's plea got, a terse 'sucks to your ass-mar'.

This particular pantomime didn't appeal much so I hit the putt thinking let's wait and maybe something good will happen in a few moments. Of course the putt went in. It never looked like missing. All square and shake hands. Thanks for the game.

Ella never found out and we were solvent enough to enjoy beautiful Cape Town. It did make me think hard, but I clung on to the idea that if there was just a chance and over-excessive caution led me to abandon it as a might-have-been that was treating luck with disrespect. Don't expect too much but don't despair too soon. All we are saying is give luck a chance.

We embarked on the *Edinburgh Castle* for the long journey back to England which was not unpleasant apart from one extremely violent incident. Much of my childhood was in the tough war-time forties when little lads scrapping with one another was a frequent and seemingly mandatory part of life. Indeed my primary school had boxing as one of its sporting activities, nor did anyone find this unusual. There was no reluctance whatsoever among that generation to settle differences with fisticuffs. I had infamously disregarded the etiquette in my clash with Micky Gent, but had received a monumental and well-deserved thumping as a mouthy sixteen-year-old imprudent enough to take on a strapping farm-worker. In my years at secondary school football and cricket were far too absorbing for boxing to receive even a cursory glance. However at Cambridge one of my closest friends persuaded me to go regularly to the university's boxing gymnasium: then in my first ever teaching post, the one in Nottingham, on several evenings I found myself alone and at a loose end. I should have been preparing lessons and correcting my pupils' work but had not yet realised how crucial this activity was and to fill in time I wandered down to the nearby boxing club. It was a fascinating place, dark and shadowy with here and there cones of light, the largest one illuminating the main ring, smaller shafts over the punch-bags. Clouds of smoke eddied under the ceiling in grey swirls, just as one saw and unthinkingly inhaled in cinemas in those days. The head coach was a boxing purist, much inclined to define the sport as the noble art of self-defence. He liked to compare boxing with fencing. 'Fencers aren't trying to stab anyone,' he would say. 'They are artists.' His name was Hal Frazier, a serious-minded Scot, and I recall him well, particularly when he lectured me about commitment. 'You know what you're doing, more or less,' he said once, and his words have stayed with me, 'but you're not committed. I've got a feeling you're the same as a teacher.' He was right and on other things too, such as altercations in pubs or on the street. 'Don't get involved,' said Hal, 'it's embarrassing and the wrong people get hurt.'

It was good advice. In the second of my Essex posts I managed to upset a pupil who threatened me with retribution from, according to him, a gang-lord in North London, who also happened to be his father. Dismissing this unlikely threat and with the throbbing headache that I always had on Friday afternoons, not an unusual phenomenon for young harassed teachers, I was walking back through a crowded street-market to my landlady's place when a car slowed nearby. In the passenger seat was a fair possibility of a gang-lord, at least until he got out. A universe so strange that I was loath to be any part of it began to take shape.

'I'm going to give you some of what you gave my lad Wyatt!' he said. The boy concerned was Wyatt Gilbert, a name of more distinction than he merited.

'You mean you're going to explain to me that a sentence needs a verb.'

'You clever bastard!' he said, or some equally witty riposte and closed in throwing a volley of punches, amid a crowd of shoppers now either pressing closer to see better this unlikely entertainment or simply bewildered by the idiocy of it all. You see he was a dwarf. How he came to be a gang-lord is hard to imagine, though certainly he had a minder, or what I took for one, in the obligatory dark glasses, still fortunately sitting in the car.

Perhaps there could have been some dignified outcome though none occurred at the time, so I pushed the little man back with my hand on his forehead as he flailed away at the air. The crowd was thickening rapidly around us, with shouts of the nature of 'Eh, look, there's a bloke beating up a dwarf.' In a sudden flash of sanity I turned and pushed away through the milling spectators. Several on the fringes shouted variations of 'What's going on?' and I recall arousing their expectations by yelling as I fled, 'There's a bloke back there beating up a dwarf!'

The voyage back to Southampton was interesting in that there were magnificent waves and often albatrosses hanging effortlessly on huge wings above the ship, recalling inevitably the Ancient Mariner shooting the albatross and his shipmates hanging it around his neck, instead of taking the sensible option of throwing him overboard.

Another diversion was a South African boxing team, presumably heading to some tournament in Europe. They sparred for hours on one of the decks, their skills enjoyable to watch. In the Bay of Biscay the waves grew turbulent and the ship pitched and rolled. The children were uncomfortable and uneasy. Madeleine, who rarely cried, was often in tears. On the day in question I came back to the cabin to find Ella sobbing and the children clinging close to her. Through tears she told me that one of the boxers from the adjacent cabin had appeared in the doorway and yelled abuse at her, saying that she shouldn't have had children if she couldn't care for them properly and when was he going to get a decent night's sleep with all the wailing.

As I write this I am a frail elderly gentleman but then it was very different. Weighing in at 178 pounds, I had never been fitter before or since and was hardened by three years of ultra-physical Southern African rugby. Now and again I still think of those Afrikaner back-row forwards, one of whom had torn my shoulder out of its socket in a tackle. In a cold fury I went into the next-door cabin. Inside were, presumably, three of the boxing team, two small men no more than bantamweights and a fattish individual perched on the arm of a sofa. One of the smaller two slipped past me and away and the other hung around in the doorway. The beefy man didn't bother to move.

'Are you the jerk who made my wife cry?' I said.

'Silly bitch, she should learn to keep those kids quiet.'

'That's your opinion is it?'

'Look at you,' he said, relaxed and laughing. 'You're trembling.'

I don't think I was but I do know the punch was a right cross and it hit him flush where the jawbone meets the ear and the impact flung him off his seat and down in a corner of the cabin. The events thus far are a perfect eidetic memory, every detail exact. From time to time I like to revisit it. The memory ends there as the red mist came down and nothing registered, nothing at all, until suddenly, just as if recovering from an anaesthetic after an operation, I began to see normally. One of the small boxers was clinging to my shoulders as if being piggy-backed, two others whom I had never seen before were holding my arms. The room was filling with people and a confusion of shouting. Eventually an older man who turned out to be the team manager asked me to go outside and tell my side of the story. This I did and he shook his head. 'The man is a menace,' he said. 'Let me go and apologise to your wife.'

It more or less fizzled out after that leaving me with an amnesiac void of what happened after the first punch. One of the bantamweights when we met on deck did add a comment, as far as I could interpret his heavy Afrikaans.

'Eh, rooinek, what would the Marquess of Queensberry have said!'

'About what?' I said.

'Well, kicking isn't in the Marquess's rules.'

'I can't remember that.' Nor could I, not a shadow of it.

'He's been asking for it for months. You should have kicked him harder. Sorry about your wife.'

Ella was full of approval. Nothing else mattered. As always.

XIII

My father was waiting on Southampton dock. We had two suitcases and that was it. The sanctions in Rhodesia meant we brought nothing out and were almost penniless. But we had a kaleidoscope of memories, two fine children and one another. In no time my mother had used her ecclesiastical sway to find a house. It was in Washingborough, the adjacent village to Heighington, and only a twenty-minute walk to my parents' place. It was a two-up, two-down sort of extension of the village rectory, itself a rambling antiquated building. Our landlord, the rector, was a remarkably vague and otherworldly man. Though we lived in a wing of his house he seemed blissfully unaware of who I was.

'Ah, I see you're admiring our cross,' he said to me once.

'Well, yes.' In fact I'd just emerged from part of his own house.

'Are you with a touring party?'

It was tempting to say, 'Indeed I am, sir. I hail from the sovereign state of Ohio. The Buckeye state, sir!' In fact, of course, with a vague gesture I mumbled something about living over there.

'Here? In the rectory! Do you really?'

My mother, who was always au fait with the intricacies of the regulation of the Anglican Church, once explained to me that he was a rector with an incumbency, thus pretty much answering to no-one (except perhaps the Lord himself, which is how it should be.) He also owned the glebe, a farm which came with his appointment. A couple of times as a boy, I and my father had helped him pick fruit on the glebe, which was a strange eerie place in the deep fenland, where all the apples were the deepest green and there was always the sound of water trickling.

His sermons were nothing if not original, at least I found them so. One was conducted almost entirely in classical Greek and another explained the long-forgotten heresy of Catharism. His congregation seemed to take a modest pleasure in the rector's scholarship. Ella, who was used to the charismatic fervour of St Mark's in Lincoln, said she found it soothing, and enjoyed hearing of the miracle of the Virgin Mary making an appearance in 1061 in the small Norfolk village of Walsingham. I found it soothing not to have to pray for the latest progressive fetish, nor to have to chant hare krishna, or listen to sermons in Esperanto.

Within thirty yards of our house were the village church and churchyard and outside our front and only door was a fine cross of remembrance for the men of the village who never came back from World War I. Ella's ashes now lie in that churchyard. Mine will mingle with hers. My parents lie only a few steps away and there are generations of Roes and Curtises (my mother's family) whose tablets and tombstones give one a sense of being part of a company from long-ago. The past is close. Very close. The convolvulus climbs over my grandmothers' graves. Their husbands died years before them. They were both busy ladies but I know how they felt when the day was over:

... when sleep comes to close each
difficult day,
When night gives pause to the long
watch I keep
And all my bonds I must needs
loose apart,
Must doff my will as raiment laid
away –
With the first dream that comes
with the first sleep
I run, I run, I am gathered to thy
heart.

Our wing of the rectory was dilapidated and cobwebbed bringing to mind at once Satis House, Miss Havisham's rickety mansion in *Great Expectations.* In the eight months we lived there Ella worked wonders, though we never did get glass in Christopher's bedroom windows and starlings kept him company at night. Of the two downstairs rooms the kitchen soon became functional and our living room was as comfortable a room as any we ever owned. The walls were two feet thick and gave it a hobbit-like snugness. How Ella made the homes she did I simply cannot say. Her financial training helped greatly and she pounced hawk-like on deals and discounts. My policy of giving her everything I earned stimulated and challenged her, particularly as it was also the exact opposite of the money arrangements of her first marriage, as we shall see in due course. Also her upbringing had made her fully aware of the Micawber principle: annual expenditure providing a profit of sixpence, happiness; annual expenditure with a debit of sixpence, misery. In fact Wilkins Micawber was unable to enact this principle and was incarcerated in a debtors' jail. He did much better after emigrating to Australia, where he became a bank manager and magistrate. Possibly Ella had similar hopes for me as an emigrant.

She did like cash in hand or in her purse. Once, as we sat together in Adelaide cathedral, I leaned towards the passing collection box only to have a twenty-dollar note whisked out of my hand and a ten-dollar note neatly substituted. 'The children must eat,' she said sternly. On another occasion my daughter Madeleine and I left Ella in the Adelaide Casino restaurant and sneaked out to the roulette wheels. Ten dollars on red became twenty and another red saw forty sitting there. 'Let it ride,' said my daughter, a bad influence in casinos. 'We're on a roll.' The ball was ricocheting around in its fascinating bouncy orbit when our stake was snatched off the table.

'Madam, thank you, the bets have been placed.'

'Nonsense,' said my wife picking up our, though now her, cash and flouncing off back to the restaurant. At least she didn't say (well, not that time anyway): 'The customer is always right.'

Teaching had to resume, however, and in one of those odd ways chance operates I got two appointments on the same day. One was for a temporary stint in Scunthorpe, the other for a permanent position starting in August back at Clee where the headmaster apparently needed an extra batsman in his cricket team. I don't say this frivolously and will consider his headmastership later.

The Scunthorpe position was the least satisfactory in my educational safari. It felt flat, like a fizzy drink open too long. Sometimes a mediocre staff will generate this semi-inertia in a school but this was not the reason. At least five of my colleagues were excellent and it doesn't need many more to invigorate staffroom and classroom alike.

The pupils were unusual. They were difficult to stimulate and gave the impression they were there because education was legally enforced, its purpose being to while away the time. Their speech was mildly disconcerting being more than usually glottally stopped, so while 'letter' became 'le'er', Scunthorpe became 'Scun'orpe' and 'weather' was 'wea'er'. My instinct said this dialect was non-Lincolnshire, which may well have been both true and false. Many of the pupils came from the Isle of Axholme, which was not an island but a strange sunken area cut off from its own county by the river Trent and famous for sugar-beet and the Wesley brothers. John Wesley, of course, founded Methodism. His brother Charles actually wrote six thousand hymns, including *Hark the Herald Angels Sing,* and the two brothers were part of nineteen siblings. My father was a die-hard Methodist and told me that, generations back, the Roe family had farmed on the edge of the Isle of Axholme. However he had no problem with the letter 't' nor did I. Because I belonged to a plethora of sporting clubs I often found myself at quiz nights. Ella usually came along and would answer the sensible questions, leaving the outlandish ones, e.g. the Wesley family, to me. She liked winning.

So much for trivia. Less trivial was seeing the research connecting smoking with cancer. Promptly I gave it up. Ella, more sensibly, had never really started, had smoked very few cigarettes in her life and even then using a voguish cigarette holder, for she was always at the cutting edge of fashion. 1967, the year of our return to England, saw constant change and not least in dress, notably the appearance of mini-skirts. She disapproved of them as adolescent though it didn't stop her wearing them. I'm certain the male half of Washingborough approved, though the rector may not have noticed.

However her full attention was focused, laser-like, on our children as they began to develop their own personalities. Christopher, being three, was able to climb up the steps of the Cross of Remembrance but Madeleine, unable to manage the difficult first step, would stand there in a fury until her consoling mother emerged. My daughter's red hair had changed to a dashing blonde, but she had all of her mother's temper and stubbornness.

You may have deduced that it would be satisfying, indeed a delight, for me to produce an account of every breath my wife took. This surfeit would, one imagines, require a deal of reader tolerance. But allow me two cameos, again eidetic memories, imprinted forever in my mind and, as she told me, one of them also in hers.

Writing this story is almost entirely a matter of remembering. Memory is an elusive quality and far from foolproof. My own memory patterns are almost always eidetic. That is they are visual, a picture isolated from the events or phenomena that occurred before or even moments after the memory. Thus one can only reconstruct limited dialogue, as was the case in the confrontation on the *Edinburgh Castle,* drawn from within a brief image. Generally this has been the modus operandi in my writing. There must have been thousands of games, usually football, cricket or golf, that formed part of my life. Most have gone forever but of the few within recall it is never the ebb and flow of the contest that remains but only a static picture and usually only one. My very first game of senior football was as a fifteen-year-old and the memory is restricted to a sort of kinaesthetic image of myself jumping high to head the ball away from our goal. I'm looking at it now: our shirts are red and black, the opposition in yellow, we are at Heighington, playing towards the railway station end, the grass is a parched brown as it had been a hot dry August, even the ball itself a similar colour. Having looked briefly at my 'photographic slide' I put it away for another day. Unlike actual slides it will not fade. Another please, one of my favourites: Christmas Eve 1968: midnight mass has come and gone and

Ella and I walk back from Washingborough church to where we and the children are staying for Christmas with my parents. About two hundred yards of our walk is through a wood, its oak, ash and hornbeam arching over a narrow bitumen path dusted with new-fallen snow. Owls are calling and behind us is the ringing of bells. Snow is hesitating down, eddying gently, just starting to settle underfoot. Snowflakes that have settled in her hair have become half-melted droplets, tiara-like, and her eyes are blue crystal.

'I hope the children are asleep,' she said. 'I've got some nice things for their stockings.'

Sometimes joy is unalloyed. The trick is to remember it.

That spring and summer slipped by. The fact that I was now Head of the English department at Clee (though not taking up my position until August) meant re-thinking my responsibilities as a schoolteacher and a husband. The latter was the more immediate. Where would we live? How flimsy were our finances? Unexpected aid came from the *Lincolnshire Echo*, which hitherto had not endeared itself to me by reporting me as a small-time habitual offender. Amongst its advertisements for housing was a one-line statement: 'House for sale, Grasby, Lincolnshire, £2000.' Where was Grasby? I'd never heard of it but it had the right suffix. 'By' sounded like the northeast of Lincolnshire, the mighty Danelaw itself, as Betjeman knew:

> Kirkby with
> Muckby-cum-Sparrowby-cum-Spinx
> Is down a long lane in the county
> of Lincs
> And often on Wednesdays,
> well-harnessed and spruce
> I would drive into Wiss over
> Winderby sluice.
> A whacking great sunset bathed
> level and drain
> From Kirkby with Muckby to
> Beckby-on-Bain.

A road-map told us Grasby could not be better placed, near enough to Grimsby and work, far enough not to be a dormitory suburb. Ella and I drove out there that same evening. Arriving at Caistor we turned north along a road which hung on the western edge of the wolds taking us through Clixby to Grasby and, had we continued, ahead lay Owmby, Searby, Somerby, Bigby and Barnetby, the villages all set on the spring-line. As we drove there were sweeping views of the country to the west, a vast plain patched with woods, fields and farms, that in the evening light was fading into blueness on an horizon fifty miles away.

The house's owner, an elderly farm-worker, showed us around. Our early impression was of dilapidation and neglect but there were positive factors too. The house was tall and set on rising land, providing views we had already admired. I was watching Ella, wishing her to like it, but so far she seemed unenthused, having observed a dozen chickens were accommodated in one of its rooms. The garden was big but looked as if tank manoeuvres had recently taken place there, as it was churned and pitted where an excavator had uprooted a whole orchard of apple trees. The septic tank or pit was near the back door and both open and overflowing.

'What do you think?'

'It's time we owned our own house,' she said.

The next day my father drove out to the house and examined it with his master-builder's eye. On his return he handed Ella two thousand pounds. 'Buy it,' he said. She burst into tears. Nor was my father finished. He delegated one of his truckies to take our furniture, what there was of it, from the rectory to Grasby, the children staying behind as it was late. We got there about eight in the evening and dumped most of our stuff into the chickens' place, they having disappeared. Our bed went upstairs and we placed two chairs in the living room. Ella lit a fire in the grate, promptly filling the room with smoke. When I poked a stick up the chimney a landslide of soot doused the fire and several dead bats fell into the hearth.

'Goodness gracious!' she said and perhaps feeling this was too Jane Austenish a response added, 'What's bloody next!' which was most unlike her but eminently excusable. Though clearly a rhetorical question, silence seemed not a response.

'I don't know, dear.'

'Falling into the septic tank?' she surmised.

'I hope not, dear.'

Doubtless the conversation was not verbatim but it would be fairly close. What was very close was one of my flashes of exact memory, frozen in brevity and clarity. We had placed the chairs either side of the fire and were wordlessly contemplating a few feeble flames consuming the bats when we realised we were not alone. Six or seven mice had formed an amicable semicircle, they too gazing into the fire.

Ella rose: 'We shall go to bed now,' she said, 'and you will put your arms around me. The mice will stay here.' As we climbed the echoing carpetless stairs she solved the problem neatly: 'Until we get a cat.'

So very soon we were part of this rural community and very interesting people they were. The village was small and compact, nor did it lie on any major road. Most people seemed to work on the land or in a rural occupation, such as a blacksmith just along the road from us. The village had a primary school so our children would need to walk only a small distance. But they were too young for school so far and they played cheerfully under their mother's protective eye. She was in her element, engrossed in her children and defining their personalities with her love and care. We acquired our very first television set and I grew used to coming home to find the three of them watching 'Magic Roundabout' before bedtime. It would be hard to identify Ella's happiest years but those at Grasby would certainly be among them.

Now I found myself back at Clee Grammar as its senior English master, which put a new complexion on things. The old make-it-up-as-you-go approach might have to become more methodical, but happily there were a number of sound teachers in the department and three more were soon recruited, of whom two were scholarly and personable men well able to teach at any level. The third was a wild card, young, outspoken and an utterly dedicated supporter of Grimsby Town

FC, who actually edited their fans' magazine. The headmaster was preoccupied with his cricket eleven and any candidature was viewed, favourably or otherwise, by what the applicant could bring to the team.

'This young fellow,' said the headmaster, 'what does he do?'

'Middle order batsman,' I said, being well-prepared and wanting the appointment to go through.

'Good, can't have enough of them.'

Plowsy, as my young protégé was known, drove a huge motorcycle to work and generally taught in a bright red sweater with a large tattered hole in it. Far more importantly he was a devotee of Dickens, was inclined to read ghost stories to his classes and did Dracula impersonations. He reminded me of myself several years earlier.

However this is not really my odyssey. It is Ella's. She was part of what happened in school, not least because she made several close friends among my colleagues and their wives. One friendship is worthy of mention. Norman, our dour and crusty Head of Languages, seemingly a life-long bachelor, suddenly married Sheila, a young, lively and pretty widow as extrovert as Norman was not. Ella and Sheila became immediate friends and the Smiths were excellent company, not least when some years later they stayed with us in Adelaide. On visiting the Cleland Wildlife Park both ladies chose to wander among the wallabies in expensive shoes and fashionable suits, neither having any inclination towards what my wife called 'backpacker outfits'.

Some years later we arranged to meet Sheila in Grimsby on one of our England visits. Sadly she was a widow again and in a confusing phone conversation gave me her address at what seemed to be a local hotel. We hoped to take her out for lunch but were surprised when the receptionist advised us that Sheila should not stay out more than about an hour. How we spent our day seemed no business of a receptionist, though I didn't say so.

We had lunch at a hotel. This time, of course, it actually was a hotel. Things went wrong in the saddest way. Sheila's old sparkle was absent, her conversation almost unintelligible and delivered in a mumble. After eating her main course rapidly, leaving me and Ella with plates still almost full, she switched my plate for her empty one and ate what was there. Any conversation had sputtered out into something like:

'The rain's getting heavier.'

'Yes, it's heavier now than it was earlier.'

We took Sheila back and went inside with her, mouthing the usual unrealistic banalities about hoping to get together again soon, holding her hand and wondering where the party-girl had gone who enlivened the evenings by singing:

Where the desert sand is nice and sandy, I'll be full of grit,
You won't see my heels for the dust!

I had not quite exhausted my clichés but came up with, 'I have to be going now, Sheila.' She clutched at my coat and began to sob. It doesn't bear thinking about. Decades later it dawned upon me that the demon itself had ridden in our car, had had lunch with us and was doubtless smugly pleased at my incomprehension and impotence alike.

XIV

Ella immersed herself in village life. She began to renovate, a skill she had acquired in her first marriage. In no time the crumbly red brick of our house was covered by white stucco and new windows were installed. The chickens' room became a sewing room. The family room, where the mice lived before a cat was recruited, was repeatedly stripped of its wallpaper. Country folk, we learned, traditionally left layer upon layer of wallpaper, and my wife insisted she had scraped off twelve such coverings. She made friends quickly in the village as various people arrived to see and admire the transformation. Our address was Clixby Lane, a tiny road that petered out after about five houses, most with elderly owners. Our next-door neighbour, a widower, had in 1916 been one of the men who dug the huge mines that exploded under the German trenches on the blood-soaked first morning of the battle of the Somme. The explosions could he heard in London. I'm sure he was glad to be back in Grasby. Three elderly brothers further down the lane spoke a Lincolnshire dialect that was at times to me incomprehensible. So that you get some idea of it here's a verse of one of Tennyson's dialect poems about a farmer listening to a sermon in church:

> *An I hallus coom'd to 's choorch*
> *afoor moy Sally wur deäd*
> *An 'eäed 'um a bumming away*
> *loike a buzzard-clock* ower my*
> *'eäd,*
> *An' I niver know'd what a meän'd*
> *but I thowt a 'ad summut to saäy,*
> *An' I thowt a said whot a owt to*
> *'a said an' I coom'd away.*

* cockchafer beetle

It sounded not unlike the Washingborough rector and his congregation, notably the third line.

Grasby had a theatrical group called The Grasby Toppers, children who acted in an annual play performing it both in their own village and in several others nearby. Traditionally a village lady was asked to direct the show, each year a different person. Ella's turn came around and her professional approach (remember Mrs Maclean's Concert Party) was no surprise. The chosen play was *Snow White* with elves as well as dwarfs because of the preponderance of small girls in the cast. She prepared it thoroughly and by the book, though clashing at times with the show's impresario, Mr Albert, an eccentric and likeable local farmer who more or less ran the Toppers. He favoured a rustic-pastoral approach on the lines of:

'Oi've got a big marrow, Ted!'
''ave you, you're lucky, 'erbert!'

Ella attempted to delete or at least dilute these and similar lines, but it wasn't easy when generally they were impromptu parts of a sort of sub-plot based on local gossip. She did certainly reduce their frequency. Mr Albert's son, the play's electrician, made one sudden appearance on stage, just as Snow White was about to burst into song, to announce that pulling the chain in the lavatory would cause the stage lights to dim or expire. The lead soprano and the elves, including Madeleine, sang on bravely as the audience pondered this caveat.

When we got home Ella was frustrated. 'I tried so hard,' she said, 'and it turned into a...'

'The Benny Hill Show?' I suggested.

'Well, hardly, thank heaven.'

'Ella, listen,' I said. 'I'm sure they've been acting plays in this village for centuries: Bible stories, Robin Hood, St George and the Dragon. The school will have its nativity play at Christmas. You're part of a long and worthwhile tradition.'

'What about the marrows?'

'They're part of it too. Just about indispensable. It was a great show. I'm proud of you.'

It was and I was. She could do no wrong.

'Mirror, mirror on the wall
Who is the fairest of them all?'

Ella's success in show-biz gave her a moral superiority where contributing to village life was concerned, but my time would come (not that I knew or expected it). Living in the north-east meant long trips back to my home football club both for matches and training. In a February match that year, 1969, on a frozen pitch, my feet had been swept away in a tackle and with what is known balletically as a *grand jeté* I landed face-first in ice-bound mud, losing three teeth, all upper incisors. On the following Monday at school the boys were jubilant.

'Sir, you can do a double act with Mr Plowes. You know, Draclea, sir.'

'It's Dracula.'

'That's right, sir, Draclea.'

My wife was, you may say, sympathetic, while pointing out that the gap included the crowned tooth so now I need not fear embarrassing the Queen if it hopped out (as it had in my Nottingham class) while we were in conversation.

When I protested the absurdity of this she brushed it aside as not to be taken literally. Perhaps she meant any member of any royal family from HM herself to the reigning Ashanti monarch, or for that matter any easily embarrassed member of the human race.

Sometime in April that year my wife remarked casually, 'Have you thought about looking at Caistor?' Caistor was the only town anywhere near Grasby, but the question itself was so out of left field as to be either prepared in advance or simply weird, like had one thought about the surface temperature of Mercury.

'No,' I hesitated. 'Well, not yet.'

'I've been speaking to Gerald. He says you should go and look.' Gerald, a local and gossipy resident, whom fortunately I liked, found Ella glamorous and polite enough to give his ideas an audience.

'Why?'

'Because I told him you'd been an important coach.'

'I suppose he means look at the football club, rather than the municipality. Tell him I was an insignificant hanger-on to a very good coach.'

It was, as so often with an Ella plan, blessed with a happy outcome after a slow start. I went to Caistor Town FC's match and an extravagant affair it was. They had abundant ability and several high-quality players most of whom seemed to be called Baffer and Bomber and so on, rather like the dwarves in *The Hobbit.* They lost 6–3 barely bothering, or indeed deigning, to defend. The coach who presumably had been primed by Gerald, asked what I thought of the game.

'Perhaps if you tried defending.'

'Would you play? There's only one match left.'

If Ella could do the pantomime this should be all right. Not a piece of cake, but all right.

The final match was at Caistor again. I've never run farther or harder with so little effect. Score 4–4.

'Look, Joe,' I said to the coach. 'Promise me you'll find three sane defenders for next season and I'll play. Another game like today will give me a coronary. Baffer and the dazzle-merchants 'll do their stuff up front.'

Ella was pleased. She was from a footballing background, her parents' house very close to Lincoln City FC's ground where she had been a regular supporter in the rowdiest section. Mrs Burley when all her children had left home became a house-mother for the club and young apprentice players lodged with her.

My wife came to watch our first game of the new season. We won 1–0 against a good side. I managed to score, my only venture into their half.

'Did you enjoy the game?' I asked, angling for what surely would be plaudits.

'It was a bit dull,' she said.

'When it's dull you win 1–0. Exciting is when you lose 6–3.' Next came a mid-week night-game, but a parents' evening at Clee ruled me out. The team lost 6–3. Honestly! It must be written down somewhere. Nevertheless by next April we'd won both the league and the county cup.

'That's it,' I said to Ella after the cup final. 'Goodbye to all that.'

'You're too old anyway.'

'Too old for what?' She started giggling. Maybe it was something I said.

There were two further consequences of my being persuaded to make a come-back. The first side-effect was rewarding, the second more like slapstick. I needed to get fitter so about four times per week I would run, either traversing the rise of the wolds or running along the road that followed the western edge. On the roadside one could look out over a black panorama lit in the vale below by occasional white lights, these on a cloudless night being only a sparse reflection of the profusion of stars above. The road was prehistoric, further south being called the Bluestone Road, though from Caistor northwards to the great grey expanse of the Humber estuary it had no name I knew. The Celtic cattlemen used it thousands of years ago to move their beasts and as I ran it was diverting to think of them, fancying that somehow, invisible below the grasses, they were responding to our shared DNA, listening and waiting for my feet to pass. Otzi, the ice-man who was found preserved in the ice of the Alps, had died 5300 years ago but in no time traces of his DNA were found in about twenty local Alpine people and no doubt there were more. I was nine inches taller and seventy pounds heavier than the ice-man so the cattle drovers would probably be little. It was hard to separate their whispering from the wind in the grass. Thousands of years later other travellers came along the ancient drovers' road and gave it a stony surface: the Roman legionaries of the IX Legio, the Hispania, who built Lincoln and Caistor too. What would their shadows say? Ella who was well versed in Latin knew: 'Ave atque vale'. After them came the Saxon and Frisian farmers and later the Danes, settling all across northern Lincolnshire as their brothers and cousins had settled around their capital of Eorvik (today's York). The ancient folk felt close as if they stirred under my running feet, yearning for the blue sky or the starry night. The presence of the past was enriching.

Then came one of my more juvenile moments. Sometimes I left the drovers' road and for a change ran eastwards over the swell of the wolds. Then the lights of the vale of Ancholme dropped out of view behind me and as wintry clouds usually hid moon and stars a primal darkness would envelop everything, not least someone in a black tracksuit with the hood up. There were few cars, perhaps one a night, and in about eight months I saw only a single person. The figure, it turned out to be a man, was cycling. He emerged from a narrow track ahead of me, turned away from me towards Grasby and was about thirty yards ahead when I tripped and fell headlong giving a sort of doleful cry, anticipating a painful fall. The cyclist at once raced away, accelerating rapidly. Unable to resist the temptation I generated a lupine howl. The rider, invisible apart from his red rear light, was soon leaving me far behind, though rather oddly ringing his bell as he sped into the darkness.

A few days later came an Ella interrogation, fraught with implication. 'Do you know anything about this story of werewolves in the hills?' Apparently the customers of the Cross Keys, Grasby's own pub, were uneasy, as well they might be at such a possibility.

'You shouldn't listen to gossip,' I said sanctimoniously. Ella, who liked gossip, scowled. 'I'll have to stop going up there,' I added. 'I mean what with the werewolves and all.'

XV

In the next six years of my teaching at Clee Grammar most of the boys were the same entertaining and rewarding personalities and so were my colleagues. But something had changed during our Rhodesian years. From a forty year retrospection it's easier to see. The sixties was a decade of change and not only in the length of skirts. Colour television had much to recommend it as did the sheer willpower and courage that took the Americans to the moon. On that morning the whole school had assembled in the main hall and, spell-bound, watched the landing. Less appealing, to me anyway, were the drug and music cultures and particularly the sanctimonious spokesmen of the decade, John Lennon and his like, who made me want to give war a chance.

The younger lads at school were still their usual cheerful selves but there was a fractiousness in some of the older boys that I had not encountered thus far. An example was their Debating Society which in the past had been a venue for light-hearted raillery and posturing but now, with topics such as the legitimacy of the Vietnam War or the damaging over-use of DDT, it had become more like a one-sided Declamatory Society, though admittedly it would have taken a skilful opposition orator to convince one of the blessings of being inundated by poisonous chemicals, be it DDT or Agent Orange.

There were signs of an urge to be non-conformist which manifested itself in everyone conforming by playing electric guitars or 'starting up a group' or wearing bandannas. Occasionally my pupils asked me for a distinctive name for their group and I drew on literature for 'Dead mockingbird' and 'Bleak mouse', though such restrained titles lacked the splendid surrealism of the Liverpool band of the eighties, 'Half man half biscuit', who produced my favourite pop song title of all time, 'All I want for Christmas is a Dukla Prague away kit.'

Having a PM like Harold Wilson was no consolation, he having less backbone and principle than a bowl of jelly and seemingly no objection to, or awareness of, the country growing steadily unlike Britain and more like an anarcho-syndicalist commune. What I didn't foresee was the impact of a Lincolnshire lady (go, my county), Margaret Thatcher of Grantham, in years to come. Nor did I foresee, and who could, that for all her courage the demon would strike Margaret down.

The Grimsby-Cleethorpes area was due for change and hardship when their famous trawler fleet began to fade into history. 1970 saw the beginning of the Cod Wars with Iceland, when the latter extended its fishing limits from four nautical miles to, eventually, a hundred miles. In the early twentieth century Grimsby was the major fishing port of the world. Yes, the whole world. After the Cod Wars the fleet faded away and now few, if any, of my pupils would tell me of how in the holidays they had sailed with their fathers to the Barents Sea or the Greenland Sea.

Somewhat against my better judgement the headmaster in 1971 persuaded me to apply for a headship. The post was close to the north-east town of Middlesbrough. Including me there were three candidates, one of whom appeared to be a deaf mute or at best an idiot savant whose special talent-field as yet remained unrevealed. The other candidate, who seemed a potential headmaster, returned from a very brief interview stony-faced and departed slamming the door. He didn't quite imitate Private Frazer of 'Dad's Army' by predicting impending doom, though he did say 'What a waste of time' in a doomed voice.

The interviewing chairman greeted me: 'Good morning, brother.' The committee too welcomed me as their brother. Was it a sort of test of my savoir-faire? Would an aspiring head-teacher chuckle understandingly and simply shake hands? Or might he say 'Hi, bro' placing himself as a soul-mate and advocate of the underprivileged. I chose the first option and waited.

'Are you not a member of a union?' I wasn't, though I did have some sympathy with unions and my brother Chris was by this time enough of a leading official of the Engineers' Union, though yet to be invited with a delegation to Downing Street for 'beer and sandwiches', where presumably any other refreshment would be unfamiliar to working-class folk.

'No, I'm not.'

'Have you ever been a member?'

'No.'

'That is surprising.'

'Is it?' I said, knowing now was the time to get up and walk out.

'Very much so.'

'Because?'

'Because you are not a member of a union.'

'I see,' I said, for want of anything better, and waited.

The chairman looked round the table. 'Are there any further questions?'

'Yes,' said someone. 'I have a question.' There was a long pause of the sort that tells one that the denouement is near, even in the theatre of the absurd.

Unable to resist, I said, 'Would you prefer to put it in writing?'

'No need. I just wondered if you were a member of a different union.'

'A union unassociated with education?'

'Yes.'

'I'm afraid not.'

'But if you were, you would tell us?'

'I would. Believe me.'

That was my quasi-interview. It probably lasted three minutes. You are entitled to doubt that but it's true. Maybe not quite three minutes.

By the time of this fiasco, 1971, we had been married about eight years and, in an intermittent and piecemeal way, Ella had told me something of her first marriage. There was never any attempt at a coherent account, nor did I ever request any information at all. She had, as was common in most of our generation, assumed that marriage would come early. Her older siblings had followed this path and the younger ones would do later. Moving out meant another bed, or part of one, available at home and one mouth fewer to feed. She told me of the unintended pressures from neighbours and friends. What girl wanted to be 'left on the shelf'? Few of her female acquaintances, and they were seen as oddities, were unmarried at twenty-two. Her husband was a Lincoln man who had been in the

RAF before leaving it on marriage; only on brief occasions of leave did Ella and he spend some time together, though so little time in fact that she missed entirely the character flaw that was to make their relationship intolerable. He was a dipsomaniac, an habitual and excessive drinker, an alcoholic, call it what you will.

She related several times the wretched sequence of events. Every evening he would go out to the nearest pub to drink for hours. Hoping that marriage meant being together she would implore him to stay at home, if only to talk or watch TV. Apparently it was all in vain and the money spent on alcohol undermined their finances, so much so that night after night she found him emptying her purse or handbag and if finding nothing, or not enough, begging her to find cash from somewhere.

She grew to dread the phone ringing to request her to retrieve him from where he had collapsed, either unconscious or incapable of thought or propriety. Day after day she washed bed linen clean of vomit and faeces.

Dreading the thought of becoming pregnant she very soon began to sleep alone behind a locked door.

Two of various squalid episodes stuck in my mind. On one occasion she drove through a storm to answer the usual sort of call to find her husband lying in a coma in an overflowing gutter, so inebriated he could neither move nor stop himself imbibing the stormwater as it flowed by. She was smart and practical enough to apply mouth to mouth resuscitation. 'This was outside the Lincoln public library,' she told me. The library's clients chose to look away, but not so her husband's drinking cronies who watched and jeered at the spectacle, as she dragged him unaided to the car.

The second incident was considerably more objectionable, not that the gutter occasion had any redeeming feature. She was woken by her locked and bolted bedroom door being kicked open and half a dozen of her husband's intoxicated drinking-mates hauling her unconscious husband in, taking off his clothes and placing him alongside her, sniggering at their bawdy escapade. My beautiful, lovely, carefully brought-up girl ran for the door and escaped through the garden and into her next-door neighbours' house. Another of our coincidences hopped up as the neighbouring lady was the sister of Derek, my bridge partner. She lost no time in calling the police. Derek related the incident to me over the cardtable but mentioned no names, so it meant little to me at the time.

'You did well to run away,' I said.

'If I hadn't I knew they would have raped me,' she said bleakly.

Eventually she began to spend more time with her mother. Though not wishing to relinquish her legal entitlement to the house she would stay there only once or twice a week. Another indignity lifted its head regarding the house: they had so little available money that her mother-in-law proposed a deal whereby she would subsidise items like the mortgage and rates if Ella renovated and cleaned her (the mother-in-law's) cottages. These were holiday homes in Mablethorpe on the austere and wind-lashed Lincolnshire coast. This meant a forty-five mile bus journey, stopping at various villages en route, then another back, and while there wallpapering, painting or simply clearing up the debris that departed tenants leave. Something half-way between blackmail and slave labour.

I asked Ella once if there was anything at all in those years that she enjoyed. 'Holidays,' she said. Twice a year she would take a week's holiday with her friends from the famous tax office, in summer to the south of France, in winter skiing in the Alps.

'Did you like skiing?' I asked, never having done it myself.

'I liked the après ski best,' she said with her giggle that meant she felt flirty and teasing. In fact one of her office friends told me my wife, between her après ski indulgences, had skied at least once down one of the main pistes at Chamonix. Nor did it surprise me.

'Did you ever think of me?' I asked hopefully but not expectantly.

'What was the point? Though I suppose I did when I spoke to your father about company tax.'

'I thought about you. And I brought you a pheasant.'

'You did, thank you. The twenties should have been the best years of my life and I wasted them. Squandered them and missed the man I should have had.'

'Did I ever meet him?'

'Idiot.'

XVI

When we arrived at Grasby our garden, the first we'd ever owned, was mostly a churned-up shambles. 'What do we do?' I asked Ella.

'A bit at a time,' she said in her common sense way. Just as well, as I had no expertise or previous interest in gardening whatever, despite playing as a child in my parents' large garden. They were both green-fingered, my father growing bountiful crops of vegetables, my mother no less accomplished with flowers. Ella's family had no garden at all; she was a city girl and I a country boy, but all the more reason to bring her the gift of beauty.

A lawn should not be too difficult and with hard work it grew well, a green carpet that climbed the slope behind the house, looking both west over the village's mossed and lichened rooftops, and east up the bare scarp of the hills behind us, where the eye always caught, just above the horizon, part of the dome and colonnades of the

Yarborough mausoleum, built aptly on an ancient Celtic burial-place. Then it was time, with the lawn as a walk for Ella and a safe playing place for the children, to learn something of flowers. Anyone can plant bulbs so hundreds of daffodils and tulips soon surrounded the lawn. The tulip had its own story: its beauty was so in demand that when, in the seventeenth century, it was brought to Europe, usually to Holland, from Turkey, there was a period of tulip mania when a single bulb cost the equivalent of a large mansion in Amsterdam. Another spectacularly beautiful plant was the dahlia, easily grown from a tuber and again with its own history, having been brought to Europe from Spain's New World empire in the eighteenth century. They were simple to grow and, the highest cachet, Ella loved them. Of course there were others and among her favourites, the daffodil, sweet pea and especially the snowdrop. Her friend Rosemary, who lived in the village, painted her a picture of a snowdrop that stood by her bedside from that day. It is still there. I was fond of Michaelmas daisies: a great clump was there when we moved in and probably had been for many years, even centuries. They needed no attention and thronged with butterflies. My mother had taught me their names as a small boy: painted ladies, peacocks, red admirals, swallowtails, the many fritillaries whom I couldn't tell apart from one another. Then there was Madame Butterfly herself, as unknowing as Puccini's heroine of the appalling future.

After Madeleine fell in the septic pit and I, fortuitously being close by, picked her out by the collar, we removed that feature of the property. There were wide parts of the garden that were almost meadow land and our elderly neighbours taught me to use a scythe, relating how, around the turn of the century, they had cut whole fields using only their scythes. Watching me cut the long grass that grew in our garden they smiled. 'It's like golf,' they who had never played golf advised me. 'Swing from the hips, keep using the whetstone.' I swung from the hips and caught the scythe on hidden stones, as grasshoppers leaped like tiny mechanical toys and little blue butterflies floated out from the long grass.

At night there were bats and moths, in the day hedgehogs ambled unconcernedly past and everywhere were bees. They lived in two hives at the highest part of the garden. A friend had given them to me. They were generally no trouble and when we harvested the honey Ella poured it into jars, for which she had designed a smart floral label, and then gave it away. On one memorable occasion the bees swarmed and she phoned me at school to ask what to do. From somewhere I recalled reading that Seneca, the Stoic philosopher, recommended beating noisily on pots and pans to convince the bees that thunder was close and they should find immediate refuge. It sounded wildly improbable, an urban myth since Seneca, who was Nero's tutor, lived in Rome. Ella and tiny Madeleine went outside and beat on pots and pans in a sort of rustic chari-vari. It worked, or perhaps the bees were tired, and my wife and daughter enticed them into a large basket, enclosing them safely with gauze. In those days the flood-tide of love and luck swept us along.

When digging I frequently came across small white pieces of baked clay, cylindrical in shape, like narrow cigarettes, an inch or two long. Eventually curiosity caused me to question one of our neighbours. He knew at once. 'They're broken bits of pipes,' he told me. 'Most country folk smoked clay pipes when I was young. I did myself and they broke easily.' The past seemed near and friendly, almost as if one could pick it up, like the fragments.

Saturday lunch-time was the theme music of *Match of the Day* and fish and chips as a big coal fire blazed. Outside, or so it seemed, it was often snowing: if it's drifting in the Wolds we'll be cut off, we thought. The village was silent and the children watched snow softly cushioning up on the windowsills. We would never grow old, we believed, would live happily in our present, lavishing on ourselves the inexhaustible bounty of time.

Oh, to think as we did then! Though to try to do so, to try to escape into the past is, we know, to re-enter a place we have doctored, its truth loaded and diluted. But how does one resist looking in at the window, even knowing that it will hurt and haunt? Just one look and walk away, for the children may see a shadow pass, though if they run outside there will be no footsteps in the snow.

My parents gave us a copy of the Lincolnshire section of the Domesday Book and we read it avidly. The Normans in the decade after 1066 had seized the land of England, the very soil, and moved its ownership to themselves. The entries in the book display an agrarian society in which the economy depends almost entirely on the fields and the labour of the men and women who work in them, the people who guide the plough and swing the scythes. They either toiled or died – not a difficult choice.

Take Grasby for example: the village had twenty-four households at that time, though how big a household was remains uncertain, but often with three generations, many children and other dependents, an average of eight people each might be too low. Even then it meant two hundred people, not many fewer than in the 1960s. The household heads consisted of six villagers, meaning owners of significant amounts of land, six smallholders owning at least some land, sixteen freemen, one miller and one priest. I know it doesn't add up but who am I to query the Domesday Book? In 1066 the lord or thane was Ulfkil, a Danish name, but by 1086 it was Bishop Odo of Bayeux, a Norman prelate.

Always the crucial element was the land. Grasby had four ploughlands, huge unfenced expanses, two ploughed by the lord's oxen and two by the village people's ploughs. It was hard labour with clumsy wheelless ploughs pulled by oxen (never by horses), eight assigned to each plough, though the ploughmen would at times use fewer than eight. An eight-ox team could plough a hundred and twenty acres twice in a year so Grasby potentially cultivated four hundred and eighty acres, though by custom one ploughland was usually left fallow.

Ella and I tried to work out the dimension and location of these big fields. The rise on which our house stood would have been unsuitable for ploughing and was very likely to have been a site for a dwelling place a thousand years ago. The church was still there but of the mill, which was also mentioned in the Norman survey, we could find nothing. There was no stream in Grasby and windmills lay in the future so it was likely to have been animal powered, probably by the oxen. I knew something of mills, having done casual work in Heighington's mill from time to time over five years. I'd also listened to a year of Professor Marsh's lectures at Cambridge and some things had stuck, for instance the fact that to buy a millstone needed a financial outlay equivalent to what a miller could earn in a year.

Where other husbands and wives converse is up to them. With us it was frequently in bed, often a sort of question and answer pattern with Ella enquiring where millstones came from and so on, when that was our topic of interest. She chose often to speculate on the role, or in her view the desperate predicament, of women in those distant days. My uncertain answers on whether the women of Grasby in the eleventh century (or just about any other century) could survive multiple pregnancies left me open to further queries of whether I'd learned anything at all at university.

'I learned it was a hard life and harder for women.'

'I'd have managed,' she said. 'I'd have married the lord of the manor.'

'What about a humble smallholder like me?'

'We could have had an affair.'

'With Ulfkil running the village that doesn't sound like a good idea.'

Both scholarly interrogation and flighty speculation were almost always carried out in bed with her pushing steadily against me on the usual pretext of keeping warm, thus managing both to fuse and confuse past and present.

'Could you move back a bit?'

'It's cold on my side.'

'Only because you don't stay there.'

'Don't you want to be near me?' she would say which effectively ended that brief exchange, because there was nothing at all, nothing, that made me happier than her presence.

I'd read Julian Barnes' novel *Flaubert's Parrot* and liked it a lot, and recently came across his reaction to his wife's death. Its impact was only too well understood.

'It makes your stomach turn, snatches the breath from you, cuts off the blood supply to the brain.'

It felt like that to me too, along with the sure and certain knowledge that I would never be happy again, unless somehow, somewhere, one fine morning, walking towards me...

The early seventies brought difficulties and hurtful decisions which were to change our lives. The central dilemma lay in the determination of the socialist government to force or persuade the various city and county authorities to adopt what came to be called the comprehensive schools system. The Minister of Education was an ideologue known as Meddling Shirley who was keen to write her name in history. It took little time: of the approximately 3600 state secondary schools only about 150 survived in their original form. Outside the state system were the public schools (misleadingly so-called) which maintained their independence but educated only about seven per cent of the children in secondary education. We will return to them later.

By their very nature comprehensive schools must be big. Most provide for 1000 to 1500 pupils and share many attributes with battery-caged chicken farming. One can argue the viability and the principle forever but history normally applies a verdict. By 2012 a majority of English secondary schools had become academies (sometimes called free schools). What their future is remains to be seen.

The news reached Clee Grammar in 1972 that it was to be amalgamated with Beacon Hill, a large and, as far as I could tell, successful secondary modern school. Not only that but the combined schools were to have a specially imported and dedicated believer in egalitarianism as headmaster of the brave new school. I've nothing against egalitarianism per se but it does seem to attract a disproportionate number of raving lunatics under its banner. Or not under it as in the case of Mrs Betjeman Lady, Ann's mother, who had more than once regretted how many of my acquaintances were indistinguishable from the proletariat. When I think of the football teams I've played for she may have had a point. An unambitious date with her daughter drew a memorable protest:

> *Don't tell me you're going, why,*
> *yes, you are,*
> *To sit with the riff-raff in the*
> *coffee bar.*

It was, of course, delivered in prose, but as a heroic couplet it was, well, heroic. Anyway most of the riff-raff had been to Winchester or Eton but in an egalitarian decade preferred to be thought of as alumni of Grunge Street Secondary Modern.

Our original headmaster, Mr Shaw, was discarded. He was far from being an ideal headmaster, in fact very far. His love of cricket was a redeeming feature, certainly, but his propensity to cane endeared him to no-one. In fact he intervened very little in the running of the school, preferring to occupy himself with totting up the school dinner money. That the school operated as well as it did was something of a mystery. It seemed to coast along, like some early twentieth century dirigible, in a disengaged leisurely way.

Our new headmaster arrived, as unprepossessing an individual as one could imagine, but clearly straight from the Meddling Shirley stable and intent on a radical realignment that would make everyone equal, an admirable enough objective so long as they are not equal last. One waited with interest to see it attempted. Our first staff meeting, at which we expected to hear the doctrine elucidated, never really got started as Steve Plowes revved his huge motorbike immediately outside our get-together, so that the room vibrated and speech of any kind was impossible to hear. I was asked, presumably being credited with some slight influence on the originator of the window-shaking thunder, to see if he would stop. He said he would do his best, which turned out to mean stopping for three minutes or so and then came further roaring. In the intervals of silence we waited, nervously tense, for the machine to restart, any rational thought paralysed.

Eventually the Harley Davidson left and we were instructed on the new vision ahead. There would be no 'discrimination' (his word, not mine) in any class. All classes would be randomly put together. I managed a doubtful interjection but was briskly informed that he had already allocated a day off for me and several other department heads to visit a school where this policy worked like a dream.

So the next day we went to Hull. My counterpart met us; he was younger than I, looked years older and had a disturbing facial tic.

'You've come to look at our unstreamed classes?' he said.

'I've been sent to see you teach one, or several, I've got all day.' I tried to sound friendly and supportive while avoiding at all costs my facial muscles going into imitative spasms.

We entered the classroom. Everyone was sitting down and behaving like sane human beings, as far as I could tell.

Any teacher will tell you that's a promising start. Certainly no-one was impersonating Dracula, though almost everyone was brandishing scissors and cheerfully slicing up newspapers.

'What's happening?' I asked, as I stood perplexed and still.

'Well, everyone cuts an article out of a newspaper and sticks it in a scrap-book and writes something about it. Just for one lesson. Everyone can do it so it's perfectly.'

'Do you have any other reading material?' I asked, trying to sound as if I endorsed the cut and paste project, while not being so crass as to mention either books or his last sentence's unorthodox conclusion.

'Reading material?'

I nearly said letters in a sequence that one can codify as words but chose the easier option, 'Yes, reading material.'

'Reading material? Perfectly,' he said. It seemed debatable which of us would have a nervous breakdown first. Probably him, as I could always either get away or do something like read the tale of Rikki-tikki-tavi to the class. That always worked.

The next day my colleagues and I reported back to Mr Sledge our doctrinaire headmaster-to-be. It seemed pointless shuffling around so I made it clear I was not a fellow-traveller on his excursion to never-never land. The novelist William Cooper described the philosophy exactly.

> As an absurdity it was so colossal that it took on the air of a great truth.

So it looked as if an appointment elsewhere was called for. I'd had a tantalising offer about a year earlier, but it was a major might-have-been, so I'd left it to simmer in my sub-conscious. We will come to it.

Lincolnshire as a county isn't flat and though the fenlands certainly are they occupy only about a quarter of its area. But the county has no mountains. When I was seventeen a friend of mine, Toby Ferry, suggested we try climbing in the Swiss Alps. Recklessly we made it up to about 11,000 feet, awed by the grandeur and exhilarated by the beauty. We were hopeless amateurs, exemplified by my dropping my sunglasses over a precipice. The consequent complete snow-blindness made for a perilous descent, worsened by my having at times to hold hands with Toby and endure the witticisms of other climbers. Coincidences have always gathered around me. Years later I introduced Toby to Ella, which turned out to be a needless formality as they had for five years attended the same primary school.

'You were lucky to catch her,' he said. I knew that, but Toby had run out of luck as most of the rest of his life was spent in mental institutions. When we learned he had been confined there we were astonished.

'Of all the people I know he seemed the least likely to suffer dementia,' said Ella.

The future can and does cast its shadow backwards.

Later, at university, I climbed again in the Alps with another friend, an entertaining companion who was a professional rugby player, an artist and later a teacher of mentally handicapped children. I was one of his pall-bearers the year he was forty.

There were other climbs in the remoteness of the Chimanimanis, and in our Grasby years I and another teacher friend ran climbing expeditions in the Pyrenees for some of our pupils. These were beautiful, unforgettable mountains, but nor will I forget two other separate incidents. I still had my ice-axe but, of course, the boys did not own such implements.

'I'll get you some ice-axes,' said Ella, with the air of 'I'll get you a jam sandwich.' A week later we had them, ten ice-axes.

'Where...?'

'The blacksmith's forge is just down the road, darling.' She would sometimes use 'darling' as a term of affection, but it could also be a synonym for 'simpleton'. I could generally work it out.

The day I got home from the second Pyrenean venture, longing to see her, she was nowhere to be found and the children were both at school. After a brief search I tried calling out, 'Ella!' and a voice from on high answered, 'Here'. The house was tall, on rising ground, the roof's pitch steep and there she was perched on the roof ridge, whitewashing the chimneys.

She had a casual indifference to risk. Several times we'd been to fairs and showgrounds and always she would be drawn to various ferris wheels and roller-coasters that would inflict switchback turns and sudden descents guaranteed to nauseate me but leave her stimulated and euphoric. Before long I declined to participate in these stomach-churning rides on the grounds they would make me spontaneously disgorge the contents of my stomach on her nice red coat.

From time to time I did go on the small train which revolved sedately and catered for the more timid three- and four-year-olds. Our own grandsons when they were that age were scandalised. 'Grandad is too old for the train,' they complained, 'and he shouldn't ring the bell.'

The prime example of my wife's fearlessness was when we were so ill-advised as to take a flight on a Sopwith Camel sort of aircraft (it still had the bullet holes from World War I) which flew into the great gorge of the mile-wide Victoria Falls. The gorge is narrow and it felt as if the plane's wing-tips were almost touching the rock-face on one side and the booming cataract on the other. She was elated, even darting from window to window as there were only ourselves and the pilot aboard. I was more concerned with the bargain I was making with God if in his mercy he would get us out of this.

We emerged eventually. I was wondering if the Falls Hotel had any really strong drink, maybe grappa or tequila, which didn't sound likely, though surely they'd have vodka.

'I'm going on the flight again. Are you coming?'

I didn't go. She did.

It wasn't the aircraft that disturbed me, or heights. Being acrophobic and then climbing mountains makes no sense. It was the claustrophobic effect of dipping into a dark and deafening gorge. Among my stories never to be read again is Edgar Allan Poe's *The Premature Burial,* and always when reading of miners trapped in pits I prayed they would escape from their entombment. The thought of pot-holing (a so-called sport) appals me. Ella feared neither height nor depth and while driving was quick to spot signs and directions. In Tasmania it was: 'Oh, look, Hastings Caves, that sounds fun,' and in NSW: 'Jenolan Caves, let's stop. Discounts for children as well.' Stoically I would accompany the family into the caverns, formulating the likely next-day headlines: 'Authorities say little hope for doomed tourists.'

You may hitherto have somehow missed my esteem for the female of the species, both individually and more or less generically, and that would be a pity. One hears little today of the Scottish poet, John Davidson, also a pity. He described his wife thus: 'She's made of flint and roses, very odd.'

Not so odd really. It described to perfection my own wife, daughter, mother, sister, Ella's mother and both my grandmothers. The name of the rose couldn't be faulted, and all of them possessed a flinty moral and physical courage.

XVII

From her grandmother Ella had picked up a thorough and practical knowledge of needlework at a very young age. When the chickens had vacated our house there was briefly a spare room which she soon commandeered as a sewing-room. Ever since marriage she had been very helpful in sewing buttons on my shirts, or mending or even tailoring shirts and trousers so rapidly that she made it seem about as difficult as knotting one's tie. My first realisation that she could operate on a commercial level, apart from producing immaculate costumes for Snow White and the dwarfs and elves, was a casual announcement that she was about to design and construct three dresses for a wedding, that is for a bride and two bridesmaids. Occasionally the ladies visited for 'trying on' but were a trifle too *de haut en bas*' being from the hunting-shooting minor gentry niche. After being told by the prospective bride that her fiancé's hunt, the Brocklesby Hounds, had failed to locate and pursue anything other than a couple of rabbits, I found myself saying, 'Oh, the poor chap.' Ella surreptitiously jabbed a needle into my thigh. The explanation came later. 'I didn't want you to say: "The poor chap, he must be heart-broken".'

'How did you know I'd say that?'

'I just know.'

Are all wives like that? Ironically when our marriage was devastated some forty years later it was because she thought she knew my mind and was terribly mistaken.

How deep superstitions run in the character is fascinating and unpredictable. My own certainty of the reality of luck, positive and negative, seemed to predicate the presence of some independent force, capable, in an indifferent casual sort of way, of giving the wheel of fortune a nudge from time to time. I expect Ulfkil, the deposed Danish lord of the manor, called this force the Norns.

Ella, in a moment of frivolity, aged about sixteen, went to a Walnut Place séance. Her description of it was comically sad. Widows asking: 'Is that you, Bernard? Knock three times if you're there' shouldn't be round a table where a mischievous red-head is knocking on the underside of the table, or trying to move the planchette on the Ouija board to provide unexpected denials to questions such as 'Are you there?' or 'Can you hear me?'

Of course, she was thrown out before long and I'm sure the board then became more co-operative.

However, despite these antics, she was quite unexpectedly a firm believer in ghosts. She described frequently her experience when staying overnight at her grandmother's house, 4 Walnut Place, she had seen a young girl walk across her bedroom before fading away. Ella had run to her granny who told her that the spirit girl came from time to time and meant no harm. She was rock-solid on this encounter, which from one so down-to-earth made me loath to disbelieve her story.

My own family were not without encounters with the inexplicable. My Aunt Annie's tale of riding in a chaise near Heighington and passing a ghost, which in her words gibbered at her (she once showed me the exact spot), would have sounded fairly gothic had she not been a hard-headed Manchester United season-ticket holder, and consequently unlikely to have a fit of the vapours.

Disappointingly I cannot relate any bona fide encounter with the shadow-world, though Heighington House had an eerie tale. The bedroom where I was born and slept in for several years was on an upstairs corridor that mystified me as a small boy. The space between my room and the next was far too long. My mother, tired of my questions, told me in a 'get used to it' tone that there was another room adjacent to mine but that it had been bricked up by my grandmother, a suicide having taken place there. Our family sold the house and the new owners chose to unblock the room and install a door. Before long there was another suicide, and as before a hanging. I recall clearly, as a teenager, walking past the house on the day of the second death and wondering why the police and the ambulance were there.

Neither my father nor my brother Chris would have registered a representative of the spirit world had it appeared before them with a written introduction. My sister, however, was different altogether, regularly encountering phantasms of various forms. It was therefore surprising when she related an incident in which some force attempted to harm both herself and her husband, unless they vacated a particular room, leaving me for once reluctant to express doubt. It had all the ring of truth.

As the children grew bigger and we acquired more possessions of one sort or another we would occasionally speculate on buying a more spacious house. Sometimes we drove through the countryside, occasionally stopping in a lukewarm sort of way at a possible alternative place. Once we drove through the marshland plain near ancient settlements like Theddlethorpe and Saltfleet, a strange, flat, lonely countryside where if one walks down little roads they tend to peter out at the grey muddy sea and one finds oneself standing among seals. It is often foggy there and was on the day we spotted a fine old farm-house for sale, standing alone among the dykes and meadows. It was open, though deserted, and we walked in. Ten seconds later Ella said: 'This is a bad place. It doesn't want us.' The children too seemed uneasy and held onto her coat. We did not stay.

She showed this perceptiveness, if that's the word, several times, always rightly. On the occasion of the potentially fatal car-crash near Kilimanjaro she walked across to our nearest neighbours in Peterhouse, the Larthe family, and told them she felt we were in danger. Our crash was exactly at that time.

A not dissimilar incident was this time in Adelaide when she phoned me at work to say she was about to fly to Tasmania.

'For any reason?' I asked.

'My daughter is ill and needs me. I know it.' She was right on both counts, of course.

It seems an idle quest to search for some explanation and equally pointless to use phrases like 'extra-sensory perception'. The incidents I've related were what they were. Tragically her razor-sharp intelligence was to fade away in her latter years, leaving her a hapless and hopeless victim, all the reason, intuition and logic that were so characteristic of her capacious mind, gone as if they had never been.

The might-have-been that my subconscious had been harbouring for about a year was itself a product of chance (and don't say there's no such thing or a tortoise may drop on your head). In July 1972 a friend asked me to be his guest at his Old Boys' dinner in Lancashire. My neighbour on one side, a man of about sixty, conversed pleasantly if rather pedantically. It turned out he was a headmaster of a school in Adelaide (Adelaide, Australia, in case you confuse it with any one of the world's nine other Adelaides) known as St Peter's College. We chatted in an inconsequential sort of way and he suggested that, if I were to write to him in a somewhat more formal fashion, there might be a position available.

'What about a short contract?' I said. 'Something like three years.'

'We could do that.' He seemed very trusting but it's surprising how many doors open when membership of the Cambridge fraternity emerges, though we did not have a secret handshake. He had been at Selwyn College (still in its infancy having been founded as recently as 1882) almost, but not quite, prompting an 'Oh, poor chap' response though it was presumptuously early to form a view on Selwyn; after another four centuries they would be cutting the mustard all right.

Mind, being a graduate of St John's, one assimilated a patrician demeanour that got one absolutely nowhere half the time, certainly not in Australia.

My Johnian friend, Harry White-Pallister, whose father owned half of Hampshire, liked to remind himself: '"Whosoever hath, to him shall be given". Says so in the Bible, John.'

'Does it really say that, Harry?'

'My dear chap, of course. Would you be so kind as to pass the port.'

Ella, as one might expect, was utterly indifferent to society's hierarchical niceties, but she did like the story of Lady Margaret Beaufort, who founded St John's. Lady Margaret had survived the murderous Wars of the Roses, had been widowed at thirteen, having already one child, later to become Henry VII. Henry VIII (Ella called him a fat ogre) was her grandson and she lived long enough to see him crowned in 1509, dying a month later. She was a very tough lady indeed and Ella, who was also a tough lady, approved of her.

But that's a diversion. I was talking about St Peter's College. We subscribed to the *Times Educational Supplement* which occasionally mentioned the school. Its reputation was good. This was just as well as my views on Australia were as uninformed and hackneyed as the next man's. Though not altogether convinced that all male Australians were named Bruce, about fifteen per cent did seem a plausible quota. The Monty Python Show's 'Bruce' skit underlined this piece of knowledge: four university lecturers all called Bruce welcome a new colleague from England.

Bruce: 'I'd like to welcome the Pommy bastard to God's own earth and remind him that we don't like stuck-up sticky-beaks here.'

Every Bruce: 'Hear, hear. Well spoken, Bruce.'

Bruce: 'Bruce here teaches classical philosophy, Bruce here teaches Hegelian philosophy, and Bruce here teaches logical positivism and is also in charge of the sheep dip.'

Ella had a robust sense of humour of which more later, but found Monty Python inexplicable. 'A man trying to eat Chichester Cathedral isn't funny,' she would say, often adding something, sotto voce, about a wasted education.

If we were to take this sizable step it would be a step in the dark (or fairly dark, we weren't after all considering moving to Burkina Faso). There would be sun and surf, Bradman, and multitudes of kangaroos and platypuses. They were all givens. There was something else, about which my Uncle Ray would often reminisce, and that was the Diggers. He had fought literally side by side with the Anzacs of World War One, and liked to tell of getting into trouble more than once with the military police and taking refuge in an

Australian camp. 'No policeman was game to follow me in there,' he would say, laughing with an old man's glee. I liked the sound of them. They even spoke the same language, more or less.

The Australians seemed to love their country and every Aussie I'd met I liked. There were some at Cambridge, and St John's had their own lad from down under. He had a sunny nature, the shaved head and hulking physique of a bouncer at some place of ill-repute, and was invariably known as Neanderthal Man.

So while there were reasons to stay it was tempting to take the plunge. Who, aged nearly forty, apart from Bilbo Baggins I suppose, gets two chances at adventure? The far side of the world!

How it seemed to Ella was hard to assess. She was an English girl through and through, she liked her home in Grasby and being near her mother, but as much as I she wanted the best possible education for her children and since the contract with St Peter's was for a three-year spell it didn't have to be a one-way trip to Botany Bay, with everyone singing 'Farewell to old England forever'.

Two of Ella's school-girl schemes were either to dance in the chorus line or to become a jazz singer. She could certainly sing and was knowledgeable on performers such as Billie Holliday or Ella Fitzgerald. About male singers she was less than enthusiastic with the notable exception of Elvis Presley. She could even do a passable imitation and if we were alone would sometimes sing in a vampish, alluring way:

> *It's now or never, come hold me tight,*
> *Kiss me, my darling, be mine tonight.*

One of my favourite Elvis pieces had the lines:

> *Yeah, it's hard to figure out*
> *What she's all about,*
> *She's a woman through and through,*
> *She's a complicated lady ...*

'Complicated' was the word all right. One never knew which persona one would wake up alongside. Often she reminded me strongly of Lizzie Bennett of *Pride and Prejudice,* though sadly, and unlike D'Arcy, I had no great estates in Derbyshire. The children were always in her mind; she had carried them in her womb and would always be there to carry them. I, she knew, was all hers, and could therefore be directed according to the Great Plan.

While the children were little, that is chiefly during our six years at Grasby, we tried and hoped to make them happy. Before writing this I asked them for reminiscences of those far-off days. Christopher refused to give any, while Madeleine painted a picture that delighted me, as it would have done her mother. 'It was truly a magical childhood,' she wrote, inundating me with memories.

November the fifth, Guy Fawkes' night: for some days before small children dragging a bogle in a pram or a trolley had appeared on our drive and sung:

Remember, remember, the fifth of November,
Gunpowder, treason and plot.

Ella put coins in their tin and gave them Turkish delight. Material for a large bonfire accumulated in our garden; when the special night came it roared into flames that drove back the blackness. Across the vale below us flared a dozen far-off bonfires. We lit rockets, sending them curving upwards into the night sky, their trajectories a rainbow arc as they mirrored other distant arcs climbing the darkness. Amid shrieks from the children bangers exploded round our feet, despite Ella's annual remonstration: 'Right, no more bangers next year.' Roman candles lit the garden vermilion. Cocoa and home-made fudge were brought out from the house and potatoes roasted in the fire's embers. And, of course, the image of Guy Fawkes burnt high on the pyre, a scarecrow figure with horizontal arms and a turnip head. On one occasion tears flowed because Ella had made too life-like a likeness and there were protests at his immolation. Another time I had to object when she clothed the effigy in my lucky jacket. This shabby article had proved itself repeatedly as a talisman. It came with us to Australia, a scruffy green corduroy jacket to be worn to football matches that we were desperate to win. Perhaps it should have been brought out in the years of the demon when our happiness and good fortune foundered, as irretrievably lost as lost Atlantis. But the jacket's flimsy magic had vaporised. Maybe it should have been burnt on the fire.

The next month came Christmas, the long-awaited essence of magic. A week or so earlier a Christmas tree was instated in the family room, its green branches frosted with silver tinsel and loaded with shiny baubles, trinkets, and little coloured lights. Above our heads hung festoons of green and red crepe. At school Madeleine made a large silver-papered star to dangle above the tree, a star so treasured that it rose for the next forty Christmases, every time to be laid up carefully for the next year. I still have it.

'Has Father Christmas come yet?' the children called from their bedrooms.

'No,' said Ella, 'and he won't come if you don't go to sleep.'

Carol singers gathered outside and sang *O little town of Bethlehem.* Ella brought the singers in for mugs of chocolate and the children, unable to sleep, came downstairs for hot mince pies. Happy among her children and our carolling neighbours in the warmth of the living room, she gripped my hand: 'You made my dreams come true.'

'Well, this...' I was about to say something trite like 'isn't a dream,' but got cut off by having the sentence finished for me, not an unusual circumstance: '...is how it was meant to be.'

Well, maybe it was. Then. But, sadly, not always.

> *The hopes and fears of all the years*
> *Are met in thee tonight.*

Christmas morning came, long-awaited, and a trove of gifts lay under the tree. My wife could wrap parcels and presents with uncanny skill, a talent acquired, she told me, in the post room of the tax office. There were presents for everyone; my present for her I had to wrap up secretly and it was consequently offered as a rather scruffy piece of brown paper that, unless watched carefully, was likely to be tossed in the waste-basket. She liked small things, tiny clocks, little silver birds or, two or three times, a diamond ring.

'Does it get any better than this?' she would say on Christmas morning, waving her hand aloft to display the ring.

Often late December, and certainly January, brought snow blowing and drifting over the wolds. Ella scattered salt on the drive to stop the car skidding. Outside the sun was pink and low in the sky. The snow reflected light upwards and crunched underfoot. Icicles hung from our roof. Snowmen appeared in the village, one on our lawn. The children gave them lumps of coal for eyes, and even hats and scarves.

Summer came in with roo-cooing wood-pigeons and, every where, bees and butterflies. Christopher rode his bike and Madeleine pedalled on her tricycle down the lane until it petered out with her stuck in a meadow. She being unable to manage the uphill slope and get back, her brother was sent to tow her home, only for our daughter to set off again with exactly the same result. Often she walked down to the Lowerys' farm to spend time with her small friend Mary, scurrying through the shoulder-high cow-parsley, trying not to be noticed by the huge but fortunately benign bull whose pasture it was. Ella was regaled with stories of how the two little girls had watched pigs and bulls castrated and told the necessity for this action. 'The males can be a nuisance,' our daughter added, quoting Mrs Lowery, nor did her mother contradict her. On the way home she liked to use the road, so that I could meet her half-way and carry her home.

Christopher and I became Grimsby Town FC supporters and in 1972 were spectators as they beat Exeter City to earn promotion. With thousands of others we ran onto the pitch to celebrate this triumph. We went walking on Helvellyn in the Lake District, but it lacked the bravura of football.

There were the usual ailments. Madeleine had attacks of croup and Ella filled the bedroom with hot steam. Our daughter also fell downstairs and broke her leg. Fortunately she and her brother avoided an impending disaster when both got into the car which was standing on our fairly steep drive. One or the other released the hand-brake and the car ran backwards, gathering speed onto the road. I saw the vehicle and passengers go past our front door and raced after them. Miraculously one or both must have tugged on the steering-wheel, and, instead of crashing into our neighbours' front wall, the car turned a neat right angle and ran on down the road. Catching it up I clung on desperately and dragged it to a halt, fortunately just before the road sloped steeply away. The gods smiled that day.

Birthdays came and went with parties for the children's friends. Madeleine's December birthday was always indoors and Chris's, in June, was usually in the garden. Several times on the June days I made a treasure hunt that took a gaggle of young boys and one small sister off through the village to find the next clue on a tree, or a gate, or even a gravestone.

While most children had lunch at school, our two ran home to have the hot meal Ella cooked almost every day. Perhaps once a fortnight she would go shopping and they would lament that they would therefore be forced to eat swede (first cousin of sugar-beet) unconvinced by their mother saying that swede was both edible and good for them. It reminded me slightly of my own experience of school dinners, when the senior boys pouring our custard would ask with studied politeness, 'One lump or two?' Though having custard poured into the pocket of one's school blazer, which happened if one was not alert, had even less to recommend it, even though the older pupils told us it was a cherished school tradition.

Grasby harvest festival was always fun, a sumptuous array of fruit and vegetables that were disposed of in a cheerful auction. We usually acquired apples and pears, though once I put in an unsuccessful bid for a giant marrow. 'Do not bid again...' said Ella.

Happily I completed the sentence, '...if you know what's good for you.'

Our lives enhanced, thinking effortlessly as one, how could we not be happy?

The memories come crowding back. Mother and daughter conspired and co-operated in making models for the competition at the local fête. One was a carousel, another the Parthenon. Both won first prize. Frequently we read to the children or told them the old fairy-tales. My tattered copy of *Grimm's Fairy Tales,* given to me in 1940, with its pictures of giants and witches, has now alarmed three generations. Madeleine recalled us 'doing the voices', which must have been such as Rumpelstiltskin or the wolf that blew down the pigs' flimsy houses before being boiled alive. Even more macabre were the Struwwelpeter stories, in which misbehaving children are used as stern examples. Augustus, for instance, refused his mother's soup so often he wasted away and died. Frederick, who mistreated animals, was savaged by 'good dog Tray', who then ate the boy's sausages while he was bedridden.

Naturally a staple reading favourite was Rupert, despite many unanswerable questions from the children such as why did Mrs Bear not make a fuss when Rupert casually went off to Japan or rode out to sea on a dragon, or how did Rupert's pipe-smoking father make a living. As to the latter we swung between his being either a middle-ranking accountant or B, i.e. head of MI6.

Ella lost her wedding ring. She dropped it in our coal-shed and it disappeared into a pile of coal and coal-dust. It took several days to find, Ella and Madeleine grubbing among the lumps of coal. I was kept unaware of this and only heard of the incident years later. They found the ring. Again the future cast its shadow back. Next time I searched for it and failed. But in the happy days there was no failing.

If anything of our idyll was omitted read Laurie Lee's *Cider with Rosie*. It's all in there.

XVIII

Our children's education worried us deeply. We hoped they would make their own way through primary school but what would be their options on reaching eleven years old? Meddling Shirley had successfully put an end to the type of school in which Ella and I had both flourished. Here and there Lincolnshire, in its usual stubborn way, had retained a few of its grammar schools but these were almost always quite small and with low numbers the variety and quality of the teachers was unlikely to reach a critical mass. The temptation, more imaginary than real, was to look for an independent school, or 'public school' in the British vernacular, but the financial outlay would have been beyond our means. In the unlikely event of somehow being able to afford it, the children, in all likelihood, would have had to become boarders and neither of us wished that to happen.

Grasby Primary School was small and homely. How long it had been there

I am unsure. Charles Tennyson, the brother of Alfred Lord Tennyson, was vicar of Grasby from 1835 to 1875 and had organised the rebuilding of the school in the mid-century. In 1968 there were about thirty-five pupils, with two teachers, one for the infants and another, the head teacher, taught the children aged about seven to eleven. With only two teachers, if both are competent, things will work, but there's a real chance the luck will run out. Christopher flourished with Mrs Vernam and Madeleine with Mrs Hallet, the ladies who taught them as infants, but the senior class was to be difficult, to put it mildly.

Our son's own view of his early schooling remains a mystery, although the village was occasionally entertained in his early days by the spectacle of his mother hauling him, protesting, to school, not unlike Shakespeare's schoolboy in *As You Like It:*

> *... the whining schoolboy, with his satchel*
> *And shining morning face, creeping like snail*
> *Unwillingly to school ...*

Once convinced of the necessity of his presence he progressed well in the infant class with, needless to say, a high-quality teacher. Things deteriorated when he moved up into the 'big room'. Our daughter remembers he was shut in a cupboard by the lady supposedly in charge; Ella went to the school to remonstrate. The incident was kept from me for several years, a wise decision on the whole. The lady concerned voiced a depressing prediction of his educational future. 'He cannot cope with an academic education,' she pontificated, or words to that effect. This was balderdash. What he needed was a proud school, full of, at worst, able teachers, but preferably gifted and dedicated ones. We could think of nothing available to us other than the prospect of St Peter's College in Adelaide. If the prospect was a mirage, so be it. But we weren't going to do nothing.

It was not a decision we took lightly, far from it. There was nothing impulsive about spending hundreds of hours weighing the benefits and drawbacks of the decision, nor was there anything capricious in moving a family and its future ten thousand miles. The Rhodesian adventure did have a slight element of caprice. Australia had none whatever.

Another factor was the future for Ella herself. What would she do when the children grew older? She had run with easy competence the national census covering the wide-spread Caistor area and both her creative and administrative skills were impressive. In a city of a million people surely there would be opportunities available for her when she decided the children were no longer what she always called 'the little ones'.

So we took the decision. Whether it was the right one, who knows? There were variables within variables. One was we were deciding for four people. Another was my own career; it had already been hinted to me that a headship was not far away. My response was ambivalent, though when was it not, except when the demi-gods of football and cricket spoke? The position of headmaster means for the incumbent, usually to his or her regret, little teaching and plenty of management and regulation. Nevertheless a capable head could be said to teach by giving a school its educational direction and a top-notch head can transform a school for the better. Only two of these doyens have come my way, though quite a number who would have got 'Seven out of ten. Well tried' had I written their reports. One of the supremos, if not the supremo, Thomas Arnold, head of Rugby School (1828–1842) was to cause national and imperial ripples throughout Queen Victoria's reign by the principles and conduct of his pupils and their sympathisers, if one excepts the notorious Harry Flashman. *Tom Brown's Schooldays* and *The Flashman Papers* will tell you all about it.

We landed at Adelaide airport on Wednesday 22nd August, 1973 and were met by the headmaster whom I'd last seen at the Old Boys' dinner in Lancashire. The day was sunny, a few cottony clouds and a sky bluer than England's, sadly, is likely to be again for a century or two at least. It had rained heavily the day before and with the Head's two sons, both schoolboys, we walked around the grounds, the grass wet underfoot. It's another of those all-encompassing but brief memory shots. Recall lasted long enough to include a number of boys training for athletics, though still being on holiday. Several came over and at once shook hands. This spontaneous action, far more widespread than in England, was appealing and remains so. For instance, with the young men I coached at football (soccer) we generally met three times a week during the season and on every occasion my hand was shaken as if I'd just made it back from a perilous ascent of Everest. Three-year-old children will do the same. I like it and miss it when I'm elsewhere.

There was a house for us, adjoining the college, and Christopher was enrolled in the prep school. Madeleine entered East Adelaide primary. I met the first of my colleagues, Mr Bruce Gordon. He was very welcoming and seemed unlikely to admonish me that Saints (as the school was invariably called) had no place for stuck-up sticky-beaks, which was a relief.

Gradually the staff and I became acquainted, or most of them as there were sixty-four in total, with only four ladies, all of whom taught in the youngest section, known as Palm House. Years later I looked down the senior school staff list and my obviously subjective judgement was that there were, in 1973, at least twenty really high-quality teachers, a remarkable proportion, and virtually no weak links at all. Much the same applied to the Prep (as we shall call it) if not better. Clearly the celestial croupier was paying out on red.

The absence of lady staff in the senior school was broken a year or two later by Mrs Chalmers. She was good value and several more school mistresses became my contemporaries later, though today there is what John Knox, the founder of Presbyterianism, would have called 'a monstrous regiment of women'. Once I pointed out to Ella that the second of Knox's three basic rules was expressed thus: 'Woman in her greatest perfection was made to serve and obey man, not to rule and command him'. However she showed no theological gravitas, or indeed any interest at all, merely saying: 'Don't be silly, and would you do the washing up.'

The school's buildings were impressive then and have become more so today, many of them of South Australia's handsome sandstone, the early architecture repeating more or less the style of the Oxbridge colleges. There was an imposing main hall dedicated to the old scholars who fought, and often died, in Australia's overseas conflicts, two quadrangles that were reminiscent of Cambridge and an attractive chapel, obviously among many other buildings. The foundation dated back to 1847 and as the first white settlers only landed in 1836 clearly education was a high priority for them. The buildings were, on the whole, centrally placed in an expanse of green turf. So architecturally and pedagogically it answered our hopes. What about the boys themselves? We'll come to them in a moment.

Ella was in her element, that is the domain of finance and administration. Bank accounts, various insurances, medical assurance, investments, were put in place with airy deftness. However the mad-hatter Whitlam government created financial chaos with inflation in 1975 and 1976 topping 15%. We had sold our Grasby property for £15,000 and brought the money with us.

'We can't have this,' said Ella. 'We need to buy land and quickly.' Our garden on the school's estate was infested by possums, which had the disturbing habit of clinging onto the fly-mesh of Madeleine's bedroom and then hissing dementedly. Reacting to this pointless behaviour we got a trap and in two days had captured six possums. Ella, soft-hearted as ever (where animals were concerned) set free the one with the baby clinging to its back. The rest I took up into the hills, driving along corrugated dust roads that brought Rhodesia to mind, even passing two grazing camels, while still being only fifteen minutes from Saints. The possums were dumped on a grassy slope, where a man was pacing out distances. We stopped and talked. He turned out to be an ex-pupil of St Peter's and a land surveyor.

'Just opening for development today,' he told me. The block looked spacious and the view magnificent. 'Fifteen thousand dollars.'

'I'll ring you back. I need to consult my financial adviser.' My adviser drove back with me the same day and was happy to purchase.

'Land never depreciates,' she said.

This was just about forty years ago so the possums presently kicking up a storm on our roof must be the great-great-great-great grandchildren of the rowdy originals I'd transported. Anyway, that's what Google says.

By the end of our first term at Saints we had made multiple friends and had a party for them in one of the school's large rooms. Parties at Saints tended, as we gradually discovered, to be generally the same, or similar, guests on a sort of unwritten roster, thus being rather anodyne. We knew nothing of this and people who had helped us in the early months got the invitations, so the headmaster came and so did the odd-jobs man, the latter actually coming from Cherry Willingham, a Lincolnshire village, no distance from Heighington.

In parenthesis, one of my hypotheses on coincidences is that movement, e.g. to another country or another profession, stirs them up. Another happened in that first term when I walked into my very first class, 5B, to see a boy whom I had been teaching at Clee only a few months earlier.

At the party someone brought out a record player and the evening turned into a dance. My wife and I were sitting out a dance, one ending in a vowel. I've already explained that such dances were too hispanic for me. A man I hadn't met, who turned out to be our bank manager, asked Ella for a dance.

'I'd like to,' she said demurely, took a ribbon out of her hair and shook loose her red tresses (she kept it long then). Her dress was black and gold. Her partner coped pretty well, considering she could have been dancing for Spain.

'What was that music called?' I asked.

'A tango.' She smiled. 'A watered-down version.'

The music struck up again. 'Is this another tango?'

'Don't be ridiculous,' she said, repeating an answer from the long-ago of our very first walk, a sort of *déjà entendu.* 'It's a fox-trot. Come on. Just do a quick-step, but slow it right down.'

'OK Terpsichore.'

We took a few steps. She was smiling up at me and I knew she held a full house, aces and kings.

'You think I don't know who Terpsichore is.'

'Most people know that,' I said, not wishing to sink without trace.

'Most people know how to do a fox-trot,' she said.

Why does one recall vividly these fleeting moments? Short of an unlikely analysis of the hippocampus, my only answer is love, the love of being alive, of being 'in the game', knowing at the time that one day it'll be your turn to go and look at the dark. And above all the sense and sensibility of loving and being loved. She had a quality difficult to name, a sort of combined know-how and delicacy. I've heard it called grace, which comes somewhere near.

She was asked to do the Bible reading in the College's chapel, the same chapel the pall-bearers were to carry her from in the December of 2015. The years have not eroded either occasion: firstly she read with a clarity that made the words sing as if no-one had ever spoken them before, then the reading was the memorable opening verses of Genesis, which later a boy spoke to me about. 'Sir, when your wife read from the Bible, she said, "The spirit of God moved upon the face of the waters" and she emphasised 'face'. Did she mean the waters reflected God's face? And why does the Bible say "face" at all?' My minimal theology was of little help though I tried to say that the bishops who translated the King James Bible were close contemporaries of Shakespeare and to them metaphor came naturally, though not usually as multifaceted as this one. I'm still thinking about it.

My own experiences of reading from the Bible to a congregation or assembly were less than satisfactory. On most occasions things started reasonably well up to 'The reading is taken from...', but the circumstances would begin to solemnise my diction into a hollow, echoing effect, like a monk trapped in a cave. Two particular notable and somewhat different readings come to mind. One was at my brother's funeral at Louth, a small town in Lincolnshire. Determined not to produce the echo effect I tried to adopt an unpretentious man-in-the-street delivery. To my surprise one of the mourners, a Johnian, another small coincidence, remarked that he had particularly enjoyed hearing the reading, appropriately from St John's Gospel, delivered in a rasping *Clancy of the Overflow* accent.

However, my nonpareil of a reading was at Shoreham Grammar in my very early teaching days. Father Kennedy, the school chaplain, asked me to read the lesson on Speech Day. Naively, though proudly, I consented. The moment came and, as I strode through the seated rows towards the lectern, it dawned on me that I had not the remotest idea what the reading was to be. Nevertheless my stride never wavered since the Bible was open, doubtless at where the reading was. Easy. Glancing down at the 'hectoring large-scale verses', hoping for a compact story or a familiar moral, there seemed no obvious one, though the word 'Moses' appeared, giving hope. 'The Lord spoke with Moses in the wilderness of Sinai...' I began, now confidently. It would be the tablets of stone, a very proper reading. It was in fact Numbers 3.14 and, thereafter, an interminable list of names: '...the sons of Gershon by their families, Amran and Izehar, Hebron and Uzziel, and the sons of Merari by their families...' On and on it went like reading the register:

'Izehar.'

'Here, sir.'

'Hebron.'

'Here, sir.'

'Uzziel.'

'Got the measles, sir.'

The audience seemed, not unreasonably, to be in a torpor. Magisterially I closed the Bible and announced, in my first-ever use of the hollow, sincere voice: 'Here endeth the reading.'

XIX

With the September to December term being, in Australia, the third and final term of the year, my classes had all had different masters for the first two-thirds of the year, and were inclined to view my arrival as either an irritant or a diversion. The younger boys were, I think, prepared to postpone their judgements for a while. Most boys entered the senior school at twelve years of age and generally left when seventeen, thus being seniors for only five years. These years were named, in order of age, Remove, Sub-inter, Intermediate, Fifth and Sixth, a mysterious nomenclature which, sadly, the school has abandoned for a drab series of numerals, ending in Year 12, that being the final year and usually the twelfth year of education. To add mild confusion, the Fifth form was, at the time we are considering, really the Fourth form, the same technicality applying to the Sixth. Confusing as it was to me, to everyone else, down to the smallest boy, that is how it was in the beginning, is now, and ever shall be. Not a problem.

There were also grades within each year and my Sixth form class was the 'A' or top class, while my Fifths were the 'B's. So they were capable enough pupils but (and this is a big but) the Sixth had been taught for two-thirds of the year by Mr Helmuth Schubert. He was a hard act to follow, having taught at Saints since 1937, retiring in December '79, when reputedly he was teaching grandchildren of his earliest pupils. I met and began to know him in the first term of the next year, he being on leave when I joined the staff. I admired him immensely. To quote from the school magazine's farewell to him, it was 'difficult to find words to pay just homage to Mr Schubert's integrity, modesty and wisdom.' In addition: 'His teaching is distinguished by the thoroughness of its preparation and the phenomenal breadth of its learning.' It was like batting after Bradman. There were two ways of looking at it: the class he bequeathed to me would indeed be well-taught, but on the other hand how would they view a Johnny-come-lately, particularly with the Sixth being in their final term preceding an important external examination.

It was a frosty reception but I hadn't come around the world to mess about and after a couple of extreme disagreements, one in each of my classes, we reached a wary *modus vivendi.* The Fifth Form, after a few harsh words early on, were very enjoyable to teach. The class had in it, among others, Tanner, the boy from Clee, and another boy whom I met long after in an Alzheimer's clinic, not for himself but, sadly, accompanying his son. This class surprised themselves, and to an extent me, by a readiness to read and, indeed, compose poetry. The 'We shoot kangaroos, not rhapsodise over them' image, which the boarders particularly liked to project, needed to be disregarded. So it was and, with an illusionist's flick of the wrist, a high proportion of them wrote poetry of an impressive finesse and spontaneity.

My own teenage efforts had usually been dedicated to local schoolgirls, though not to Ella, who would have known them for the jejune saccharine they were, her favourite poet being John Milton, from whom she could quote at length, which says it all. I needed, but never had, a teacher to steer me away from juvenile imitations of Algernon Charles Swinburne, who was responsible, for instance, for:

> *Where all days through thine hands*
> *in barren braid*
> *Were the sick flowers of secrecy*
> *and shade,*
> *Green buds of sorrow and sin and*
> *remnants grey,*
> *Sweet-smelling, pale with poison...*

and so on. These particular lines do make it into the *Oxford Book of English Verse*. Oxford! 'Home of lost causes,' according to Dr Arnold.

I taped the boys' poems on the wall, thereby producing a number of critics, though even our self-professing philistine earned some respect with verses starting:

> *Cricket, cricket, cricket all the day*
> *Cricket is the game for men to*
> *play ...*

He was pleased when told that cricket far exceeds other sports as an inspirational topic for verse. To demonstrate I recited the following:

I've been standing here at this wicket, since yesterday just arter tea,
My tally to date is eleven and the total's an' 'undred an' three;
The crowd 'as been booin' an' bawlin'; it's booed and it's bawled itself 'oarse,
But barrickin', bawlin' and booin' I takes as a matter of course,
'Oo am I to be put off my stroke, Mum, becos a few 'ooligans boos?
An Englishman's crease is 'is castle: I shall stay 'ere as long as I choose.

'That must be Boycott,' he said, recognising a long-time foe. 'Good poem though'.

Another emergent image, same class: a boy writing a few lines, eight or ten, no more, on dropping a flower onto his grandmother's coffin.

'Will you read it out to us?' I said.

'I'd rather not.'

'It's worth reading.'

'Are you sure?'

He read it aloud. There was silence. Had I got it wrong? Then a boy began to clap, then another, and gradually everyone there. Later I showed the poem to Ella. She read it and gave it back. 'He's hurting, God bless him,' she said. Forty-two years later our grandsons dropped flowers on their gran's coffin. God bless them and her.

Schubert, who was Head of English, seemed to be pleased when he returned. He told me how there had been for several years an edginess, a sort of generational discord among the older boys, which he attributed to the influence of the Vietnam War. Conscription among twenty-year-olds was compulsory in theory, but only happened if a marble holding one's birthdate was drawn out in an annual ballot, since the army required only a limited number of recruits. It sounded very like roulette and just as chancy. For instance, in the eight ballots from 1965 to 1972 my birthdate emerged only once, but my son's appeared four times, so had we been eligible we might have had different opinions on luck.

Christmas came and good reports from the children's schools so, after our big party, we set off on a journey that was to be a salutary lesson for us. 'Space is big. Really big. You just won't believe how vastly, hugely, mind-boggling big it is. I mean you may think it's a long way down the road to the chemist's, but that's just peanuts to space.' Pretty much the same applies to Australia, as Ella, the children and I realised during the journey in our Holden Belmont (a great car, by the way) to the Barrier Reef. We hadn't done much research on the Reef and probably less on the marathon required to get there. To our credit we did reach Rockhampton. The Whitsundays were still 400km in the distance and Cairns a daunting 1000km, about the same as driving from London to the French Riviera. In any case this all became academic as rain fell in deluges and, shortly after leaving Rockhampton behind, we were halted where our road was blocked by a metre-deep torrent. The children seemed to enjoy our stay there, watching an occasional vehicle foolhardily try to cross and get swept away. Despite this it was actually easy to feel an affinity for Queensland, as apparently they had initiated and fostered the sport of dwarf-throwing. We spent several days camped out in a sort of box-tent city which very soon provided a perfect example of my wife's very individual sense of humour.

She was impervious to the Monty Python absurdities. One of my favourites portrayed John Cleese playing some sort of interviewer with a microphone, leaning down to an obviously shy, small boy in school uniform and cap (Michael Palin) and asking gently, 'What's your name?'

'Eric.'

Again gently: 'Would you like to have a sixteen-tonne weight dropped on you, Eric?'

'Don't know.'

This, though only a fraction of the skit, reduced me to helpless laughter. Ella herself laughed irrepressibly in the tent city when the adjacent tent collapsed, spilling gallons of water on the head of a passing camper. This partiality for burlesque surfaced on a separate occasion later, when we did actually reach the Reef by taking the sane option of flying. A close friend dived off the ship, partly dislodging his mask enough for it to fill with water. He scrambled back on board, choking and spluttering, unable to remove the mask, not being consoled by my wife falling off a deckchair laughing. On a third occasion, this time flying back from a trip to England, a cabin attendant opened an overhead compartment and a large box fell on someone's head. Her smothered mirth (i.e. Ella's) lasted several minutes until realising that it was her box and full of valuable china, whereupon there were stern words, certainly containing the word 'compensation'.

There were some comedians whose humour she enjoyed. The Two Ronnies, Morecambe and Wise, and Tommy Cooper come to mind. Tommy died on stage at Scarborough in Yorkshire, an incident macabrely available on Google. Among the audience was my brother Chris. 'I thought it was part of his act, I couldn't believe it,' he told me, in all likelihood duplicating a passer-by in Gela, in 455BC, saying: 'Then I saw this tortoise fall on Aeschylus's head. Can you believe it?'

She was uncompromising where bawdy humour was concerned and poured contempt on the Benny Hill Show's approach. On private or social occasions if the language became either profane or coarse she would chill those involved with a sort of freezing contempt. Only between the two of us would she indulge in a conversation which if it could be called risqué was only most delicately so, and expressed in an effervescence of giggles at her own daring. I thought her lovely, which is an adjective a bit worn around the edges, but if the shoe fits ...

Australia, like space, is big. Our seemingly endless journey to Rockhampton was evidence enough. It seemed interminable as we drove; sometimes, when we got out and stretched our legs, the sky was impossibly huge and the views, of close-cropped fields stretching away, almost replicated the sky in their immense plainness. Only back in the car was there the comfort of one another and smaller objects, like the children's toys or a flask of tea. They were more our scale and more real than the mirages dancing on the road.

This reaction was certainly nothing unique. 'The outback' is a great name: it's the land out there beyond the cities, almost beyond the reach of rain, a vast emptiness, a salt lake without water, where one desert dwindles and overlaps into another, the Sturt into the Simpson into the Gibson into the Great Sandy Desert, the latter sounding as if the explorers had finally run out of names.

In the night-sky the stars were either strange, or familiar constellations distorted, Orion upside down and my favourite star, red Betelgeuse, bigger and redder. Ella even found caravanning in England an ordeal and preferred life in the city, almost any city, and liked Adelaide which had places that weren't mirages, such as shops or banks or schools, or helpful organisations like hospitals or the police. She would not have exchanged Adelaide for any English city and, if she ever yearned to be elsewhere, it would have been to some imaginary place consisting of Adelaide surrounded by the Lincolnshire countryside.

Our car-trip, basically to nowhere, reminded me of Ursula le Guin: 'It is good to have an end to journey towards; but it is the journey that matters in the end.' Le Guin was a favourite among the younger boys of my classes, they being often avid readers and writers of science fiction and fantasy.

In the long run the appalling end we were journeying towards was less of an end than misery's furthest extremity. For at least five years it was simultaneously a journey and an ending, so horrifying that the thought of still having to describe it makes me feel sick. That's when the demon makes its entry and usurps the story. That's when the fun and the laughter drain away.

1974, my first full year at Saints, saw Mr Schubert kindly give me the top English set again. They were able and attentive pupils and in their final examination produced results which Schubert gratifyingly remarked were the best he remembered. I'm fairly sure they all got A grades, which is one, but not the only, way of describing best. At the end of the year. Ella and I went on a school trip to New Zealand. This was a bus journey starting in Auckland and finishing at Milford Sound, with various stops to appreciate this beautiful country. Though Ella was the only lady on the venture she was a source of fun on the longer drives setting up, particularly for the younger boys, boisterous word-games, so that our organiser suggested, not unreasonably, that the participants might occasionally take the opportunity to watch the scenery. We visited the Southern Alps and scrambled up the lower slopes of the Franz Josef glacier. Later in the general excitement we boarded our bus and drove about fifty miles before realising Ella had been left behind. The usual bonhomie and laughter in the back of the bus had led me to believe she was there in the thick of it. On returning to the glacier, our, or more accurately my, reception was glacial.

'I remember when I was dumped in New Zealand' was a favourite dinner party reminiscence, along with a description of, as she put it, being 'abandoned' in the Karoo.

Milford Sound saw another example of my wife's schadenfreude when, on a cruise, a boy brought on deck a tray of a dozen or so mugs of coffee, just as a large wave sent our craft heeling over and him stumbling against the rails, tray and coffee cascading overboard.

'I'll have another try, Mrs Roe,' he said resolutely.

'Yes, do, Benny. I look forward to it.'

XX

There's something to be said for the commonplace and the ordinary. They are where the horror can't reach one. There are worse things than going for a hair-cut or taking the dog for a walk, for instance some malignant force wrecking my wife's brain. That's worse. A lot worse.

Perhaps I was wrong to cast doubt upon the young short-story writers of my classes, who enjoyed composing three or four page stories, usually entitled 'The Cataclysm' or 'The end of civilisation as we know it'. My criticism was that almost all the writing was devoted to a close description of getting out of bed, getting dressed, having a slice of toast, choosing between jam and marmalade, brushing teeth, before, about 8.45am, the Martians launched their invasion of Earth, this crucial event meriting only about five lines.

The more I think about it the more it seems the boys were right. The horror comes soon enough. Enjoy the marmalade. My belated apologies to 4B. Mea culpa, lads.

Sometimes in my teenage years I kept a diary, though not for long, usually after receiving one at Christmas but losing interest by April. My entries had a rhythmical reiteration of the day's structure, whereby only the obvious was painstakingly recorded: 'Got up and got dressed. Had breakfast. Went to school. Came home. Did homework. Went to bed.' Something must have happened worthy of mention but there was no entry recording: 'Hit Micky Gent on the head with a half-brick'. My fifteenth year was a red-letter adolescent year, with, briefly, a girlfriend, and my very young debut in senior soccer. Neither experience made it into my diary, certainly not usurping the space that noted I had gone to school. Indeed my diary, 1950, the only one still in existence, mentions no spectacular occasions.

Not that they did not occur, for I received a hated Saturday detention, thus missing an important match. My crime was to shriek out 'Port Vale' in the silence of a chemistry exam. Some of my fellow examinees and I had soon exhausted our knowledge of chemistry and were passing the time by compiling the names of the eighty-eight clubs in the English football leagues. We were stuck for some time on eighty-seven. When the missing name came to me it would have been better to shriek 'Eureka' and even possible to defend this as an appropriate reaction, as history tells us that Archimedes coined the expression after a successful chemistry experiment. When Mr Battersby said, 'What was that?' my friend Jimmy Bebbington, trying to find a half-rational response, came up with 'He said, "Oxygen", sir.'

'Ah-ha, cheating,' said Mr Battersby.

Somehow I couldn't bring myself to say: 'Yes, I said "Oxygen" but I meant "Port Vale"'.

It was getting close to Humpty Dumpty lecturing Alice that 'glory' also meant 'a nice knock-down argument'.

None of this entered my diary. Tedium has its own decorum.

To avoid reproducing the annual diary effect let's deal with the next thirty years in topics.

When we purchased the land on the virtually unpopulated hillside known as Skye, it boasted one house only. We waited a while before setting out to build. In 1976 Ella's patience snapped and she bought a drawing-board, rulers, set-squares, protractors and so on and sat down to design a house. This was done, though not without angst, as a survey had revealed a longish narrow ridge of rock near the top of the block. Though this was restricting it was ideal as a foundation and well-placed to ensure the view was uninterrupted. She pored over the board for several evenings and then announced: 'I set out to design a house, and I have designed a railway carriage.'

The narrow ridge had forced the shape on her but it looked fine to me. '"Striving to better, oft we mar what's well,"' I said sententiously.

'Is that Shakespeare?'

'*King Lear*,' I said. It was often an examination text.

'Just because Shakespeare says it, it doesn't mean...'

Later we got an architect to produce a plan. There seemed little, if any, difference between his and hers.

The excavators moved in and tore off the topsoil to expose the ridge, and elsewhere to produce a fairly regular slope. The drawback was evident enough. The steepness of the slope meant that on stepping out of the house one was likely to go scrambling, or even rolling, downhill. In reverse one almost needed crampons to scale the slope upwards. The only way to avert this predicament was clearly to construct terraces.

Then luck stepped in (it was still holding). Driving along Port Road I saw a notice-board: 'Stone for sale'. A house was being demolished and the contractor sold me its fine sandstone for two hundred dollars, provided the stone was removed within a week.

It looked a labour of Hercules, perhaps not as dangerous as killing or capturing various violent creatures and not as nauseating as cleaning out the vast dung-piles of the Augean Stables in a single day. This latter feat was invalidated at the time, on the excuse that Hercules, by diverting two rivers through the stables, had not actually cleaned up the ordure by hand. Clearly Hercules had not read the small print. Where my labour was concerned the timescale looked difficult.

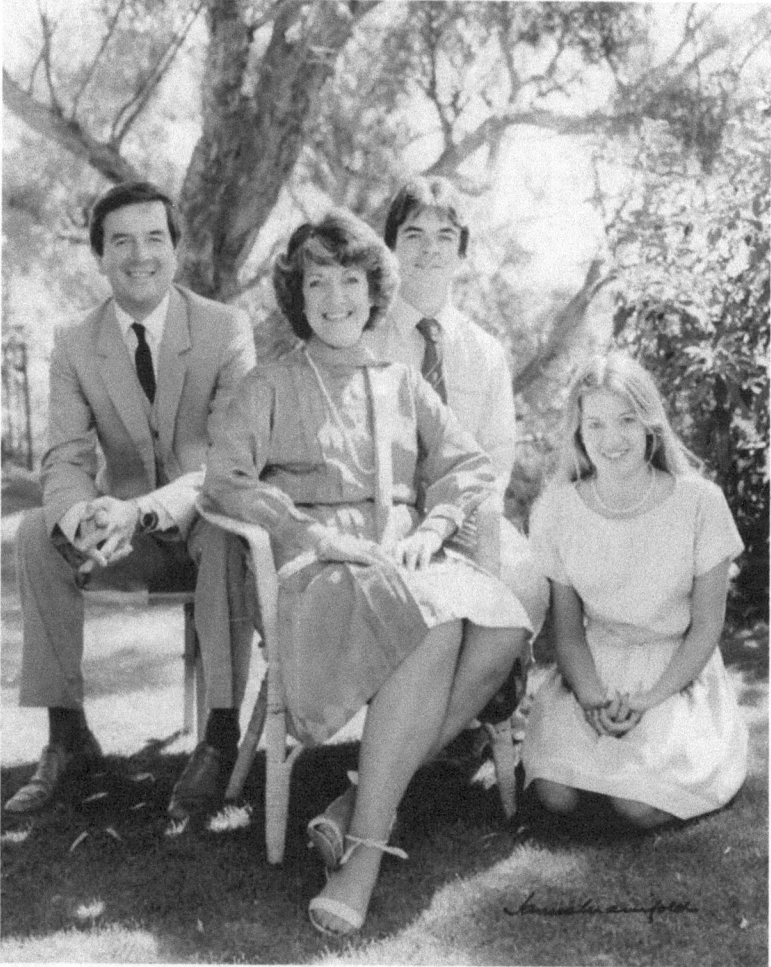

John, Ella, Christopher and Madeleine, 1983

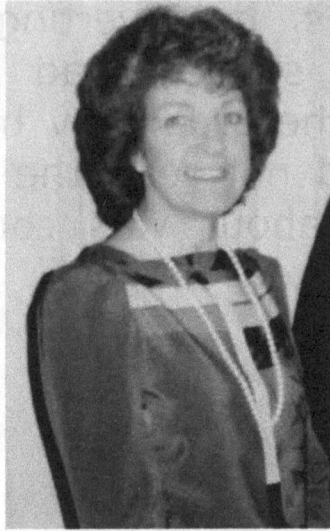

Ella, 1994

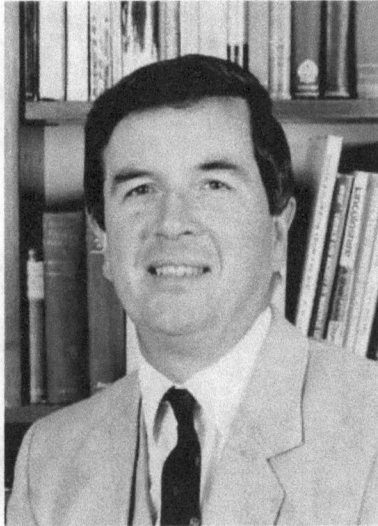

John, 1994

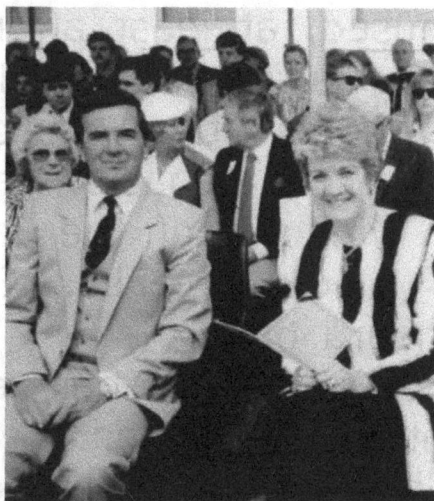

Happy parents: John and Ella at son Christopher's Passing Out Parade, Duntroon, 1986

On my side was the fact that I had a truck-driver's licence, fortunately kept up to date since my mill-hand days. My cousin and close friend, Tom, with whom I still correspond, also drove lorries for his father's firm and one day we had inadvertently brought the main street of Lincoln, pedestrians and traffic, to a standstill. This busy street ran under a stone arch and our lorry, stacked high with straw bales, would just scrape under it, or so we urged one another to believe. Inevitably our load caught the arch, strewing forty or fifty bales in all directions. Pedestrians stood bemused, at least after dodging the toppling bales, but vehicle owners and eventually the police were unforgiving. This debacle was almost under the windows of the Tax Office, but took place pre-Ella. She had, however, heard of it.

'That was us,' I told her years later.

'I might have guessed.'

To collect the sandstone I had bought I hired a truck and recruited some of the boarders. About eight or ten of them, plus Ella, drove down Port Road. The roof had gone but the walls were still erect, at least until my cheerful pupils had torn into the job, levering the walls down with crowbars and loading stones onto the truck. I shudder to think of how many by-laws and safety codes we would have broken had it been today. The truck was driven back to Saints with the boys and Ella perched high on the stones. Along North Terrace it felt like a Roman triumph. Three days later we did it all again. They were great kids, from Lock and Burra, Parachilna and Quorn, Hawker and Millicent.

We bought a concrete-mixer and built the main wall. It was hard but satisfying, and the stones looked good, honey-coloured and chiselled. As I found it difficult to work with gloves on, often my fingertips oozed blood. The wall was head-high and thirty metres long, its top course of stones exactly level with the house's lowest layer of bricks. The remaining stones formed other terraced walls about waist-high, adding another fifteen metres in length.

But the slopes were still too extreme, calling for more walls. Fortunately someone suggested slate as an easily-worked material and so it proved to be. Over the next three years were installed about a hundred metres of slate walls, again about waist-high and about a hundred metres of slate paths, plus a ninety-square metre terrace. As we did not wish to leap from one terrace to another there had to be steps. I tried to make it thirty-nine steps, as in John Buchan's novel of that name, a boyhood favourite, but eventually there were sixty. A by-product to the labour was that my weight, to my surprise, shot up. 'It's all muscle,' said Ella. 'You should go in for body-building, you could be Mr Universe.'

'Better than Mr Puniverse,' I said, quoting a term of ridicule my pupils were over-inclined to use on anyone smaller than themselves.

'I don't think I'd appreciate Mr Puniverse,' she said, teetering on the edge of propriety.

Normally maths was left to my wife who found my innumeracy amusing, so sorry about all the boring statistics. 'There are lies, damned lies, and statistics' is attributed supposedly to Benjamin d'Israeli; I wished I'd thought of it first. However if you bring a tape measure up to our place you can check it all out.

There remains a cherished memory of those days. To get our slate we used to hire a truck and many times drove up to the Wistow slate quarry, not far from Mount Barker. There we would choose the pieces of slate we wanted and fill the truck. It was invariably hot, the quarry was always dusty, often noisy with machinery. Ella, in an apron and headscarf, doing a Russian peasant impersonation, worked tirelessly. We would set off home, but always stopping at a small store that sold drinks and ice-cream. Pulling onto the verge we would eat our ice-creams in the cab. Her hair was coated with dust, despite the scarf, sweat had formed lines in the dust on her face, and the ice-cream ran down her chin.

'Do I look a mess?' she would say.

'No, you look great, missus.'

'No, I don't.' But she did, and she knew she did. 'And stop calling me missus.'

Meanwhile with both children at school and with a new house, though undecorated and relatively unfurnished, she showed a skill-set and practicality that amazed me. The house was painted, rooms were wall-papered, curtains flowed off her sewing-machine, as did quilts and bed-spreads. Miraculously she constructed furniture. The chairs and sofa of our drawing room today are as stylish and comfortable as when, forty years ago, they were made. The house's transformation took about six months. It was hard to believe then and is now.

She had done some teaching in needlework and dress-design at Norwood TAFE while we were still living at Saints and, with the house more or less as she wanted, she took a full time post there.

Now, with two incomes, the financial expertise came into play. 'Mortgages are a waste of money,' she said, and very soon we had no mortgage. She liked blue-chip shares and gradually acquired them. She built up a collection of term deposits, moving them regularly in search of higher interest rates. When we acquired a computer this became easier. She was fascinated and in no time became computer-adept, if that's the term.

When the demon struck it struck hard and centrally. It must have been reading Clausewitz. The occasion pervades my mind. Ella had brought all her financial documentation into our diningroom and placed the papers on the table. She intended to complete our tax returns, so it must have been July 2010. She was standing completely still, looking down at the pile.

'I don't know what to do,' she said.

'Well, just do it as you always have done.'

'I can't. I can't do it.'

Standing there, as if alone and lost in a thick fog, she began to cry.

She never touched our finances again. Not once. She never visited our bank or our financial adviser, never wrote another cheque or referred to the computer again. Without her I was to fumble and struggle for years. The final piece of the puzzle did not fall into place until July 13th, 2017, nineteen months after her death, when, as from nowhere, appeared $17,000, a sum which I thought existed but had been so difficult to locate I'd virtually written it off.

It was a dreadful blow for her to lose all of her natural and acquired expertise in finance, but we could weather it. The blows to come were worse by far as the demon clawed at and savaged her health, her mind, her self-respect, her beauty and her happiness.

However, back in the unforeboding seventies, Ella was constructing a future for herself. She enjoyed her work at

Norwood, and decided to study for a Degree in Education. In an identical situation I had not bothered with such a qualification, subconsciously assuming that teaching was one of those hardscrabble hands-on jobs like beet-singling. She was far more realistic, acknowledging it had to be done.

On May 3rd, 1980 she became a Bachelor of Education of Adelaide University. There's a photograph of her on the day, in her mortar-board and her ochre and blue gown, plus the customary high heels. Among her favourite films was *Top Gun;* she often sang its theme song: 'Take my breath away'. That photograph still takes my breath away.

We spoke about the degree afterwards. She saw it as a necessary step forward, but wished to take another course that would be purely for enjoyment.

'What do you have in mind?'

'There's a Diploma in Fine Arts that sounds interesting.'

She threw herself into this course with delight. It allowed her to specialise and at first she chose antique furniture, but though interesting it had less of the practical work she enjoyed. Switching to the skills and design-arts of the coppersmith, silversmith, enameller and glass-maker, every week she brought a creation home. She designed and created two stained-glass windows and installed them in our main bathroom, as well as stained-glass panels in the dining-room door. Both display stylised flowers and leaves in pink and green, so refined and elegant they still, again, take my breath away.

One of the bathroom windows was broken by our then seven-year-old grandson Alex, with a slashing square cut. He and I stared in horror.

'Baba,' as he called his grandmother, 'will come out! Shall we run away?'

'No, it won't help.'

She came: 'Who did that?' she said menacingly.

'I did, Baba.'

'There, there, never mind then.' What a relief!

A day later it was repaired with nimble-fingered ease.

In her silversmith classes she made a ring, designing a clasp that held an opal I'd once given her as a birthday present. She wore it almost permanently. In hospital, a few days before her death, I noticed that, along with her wedding ring, it was no longer there.

'Where are your rings?'

'I think someone took them off.'

My enquiries got nowhere. It may be as well, for I was murderously angry. Not finding the thief galls me to this day.

But there's plenty more to tell before we reach the bad years, the years after 2010. In 1980 the powers that be made me Housemaster of Young House, a position which terminated only with my retirement. It pleased me because their colour was red and this and luck, I knew, ran hand in hand. My school's colour was red, so was my college at Cambridge, so was my first and favourite football team; my successful come-back at Caistor Town FC, in the werewolf days, meant playing in red. Then there was my girl's glorious blood-red hair. In our closest moments, whenever we opened our hearts to one another and spoke only the truth, undecorated by jest, I called her 'Red'. No-one ever heard or knew. It was her hidden, true name, spoken only just before sleep.

Since the House was considerably younger than most other Houses they had no traditional sports shirt. Morale needed this.

'How many do you want?' said Ella.

'About eighty.'

'Badge?'

'A kookaburra.'

'OK. What about blue trim on collar and sleeves?'

'Thanks,' I said, overwhelmed.

'Sounds easy enough.'

She made them in less than a week. Already we looked competitive. Boys like winning. The natural leaders and I conferred. Our first targets were mass entry sports, notably swimming and athletics, that had points simply for attempting an event. If everyone swam or ran every event we'd be highly competitive. It even coined a phrase of honour, 'The drowning moth', awarded to any gallant little lad who tried but sank before making the distance in the butterfly event, a sort of junior stakhanovite.

I coached the House soccer and cricket teams and watched every moment of their games. Eventually we began to collect trophies. Some matches became legendary. The junior cricket side's final came down to the last two balls of a hundred over game. Needing twelve to win our last batsman swung desperately and hit a four, but the umpire called a no-ball (worth two in those days). With six needed came a swing and a miss. So now it had to be six off the last ball, with the juniors in a frenzy in the pavilion.

'Don't worry, lads,' I told them. 'We're riding the wave.' And the sixer climbed the sky.

They liked being different. For instance, there was a period of two years or so when, at morning services in Memorial Hall, the House would sing hymns with an unprecedentedly noisy gusto, causing a mild controversy, since the headmaster had several times remarked that he disliked hymns being mumbled, as he put it. Rankine and his mates, singing like a revivalist rally, remedied that. The red House liked to push the envelope.

But the icing on the cake for many was the films we made. These were unique in that they were not the usual medley of the year's events but were actually stories with a coherent if semi-demented plot. They were in turn 'James and the Giant Possum', 'Ramy builds a time-machine' and 'The Monkey God'.

The first of these produced a supreme moment when two parents and their children were walking round the school before deciding whether Saints was an appropriate forum for their children's education. Unfortunately they observed a very big boy pushing a very small boy's head into the ornamental pool near the Big Quadrangle.

'I'm all right,' said the small boy, spluttering water and brushing weed off his face. 'That's the school bully. He ducks all new boys.' Releasing no further information the little lad left. What the horrified group failed to see was our camera-man, some twenty yards away, inadvertently hidden in the

Quadrangle, taking an 'artistic' shot through an arch. Camera-men always did this sort of thing. The family chose not unreasonably to send their children elsewhere.

'The Monkey God' was our final and crowning epic. I appeared in it myself as a sort of Lord John Roxton, though fairly anonymous with a pith helmet and heavy moustache, supposedly leading an expedition to King Solomon's Mines to retrieve the Monkey God. Much of this film was shot in the valley that forms the lower part of Skye and Ella sometimes came down to watch, bemused by our antics.

Things looked grim as we approached the mines.

> Mbongo: 'Bwana, the bearers no go on. We bearers know we will all die in the Valley of the Kings.'

> Colonel: 'You're the head bearer-wallah, Mbongo. Give every bearer who will go on a ball-point pen.'

> Mbongo: 'Bwana, we go on.'

Danith Woods (our only coloured boy) was of course type-cast as chief bearer-wallah, and he, like others, amused me by playing his role absolutely straight. Another such was Matthews, playing a sort of Crimean War sergeant:

> Colonel: 'Wait till you see the whites of their eyes!'
>
> Sergeant: 'Whites of the eyes it is, sir. 'Ere, 'old yer fire, Perkins. Wait for it, lad.'

And in the final battle with the Zulus:

> Sergeant: 'The Germans have got me at last, sir.'
>
> Colonel: 'Not the Germans, sergeant. The Zulus.'
>
> Sergeant: 'That's right, sir, the German Zulus.'

For the battle itself our library ladies, usually in hysterics, did their best to insert our revelry into the film *Zulu,* notably the Battle of Rorke's Drift, which we bravely re-won. We had to borrow a Polynesian islander from the Boarding House for close-ups of the fighting, but he did well, even bringing his own ornamental spear.

Our theme tune was an inappropriately catchy song from the 1920s:

*I'm just a kid again, doing what I
did again, singing a song,
When the red, red robin comes
bob, bob bobbin' along*

I liked the tune but it took Ella to point out how apt were the words: 'You're all just a bunch of kids,' she said.

The House system had a lot going for it as, in a fairly big school where an unassuming young boy might have been submerged, his House, if properly run, was a sort of extended family.

Ella and the House Captain's mother ran, always successfully, the annual dinner. She also donated the Ella Roe Prize. After examining our prize list of various gladiatorial trophies and awards, she remarked, correctly, that the one totally neglected achievement was academic excellence. May her name be read out in perpetuity, or at least as long as the House exists.

Among the school's activities she supported, her favourite was drama and for years she was the costume mistress of various plays. *St Joan, The Importance of being Earnest* and

Midsummer Night's Dream come to mind. The latter was an alfresco production, under a starry sky, in the closeness of the Little Quadrangle, made particularly memorable by a fifteen-year-old Titania, blonde hair tangled with ivy and jasmine. 'My daughter,' said Ella for the benefit of those who could not read the programme.

It seems like yesterday that Young House's captain led the Saints First Eight to a desperate victory in the Head of the River race, splashed to the shore, picked Ella up in his arms, tripped and fell backwards. Both disappeared under the crystal waters of West Lakes, emerging to applause that if it was not universal should have been.

Naturally it wasn't all moonlight and roses. She always dealt with other ladies herself. An extremely patronising wife of one of my colleagues was so ill-advised as to condescend to my wife at some do or other. Another guest told me, gleefully, of the withering Walnut Place response.

If she ran foul of men, apart from the incident of the witchdoctor, it was delegated my way. This seemed to me right and proper and somehow satisfying. Sometimes it seemed she drove our marriage and family along, but she did so knowing she had a minder close and watching. Predicaments demanding intervention did occur a number of times. The incident on the *Edinburgh Castle* was one such. Another, which took place in the boardroom of a well-known Adelaide company, only just avoided violence when the man concerned, having absurdly suggested Ella had mishandled the funds of a cancer charity, was forced to produce a written apology, in an ugly scene that would have turned a lot uglier had he not done so. The man was 'majorly in error', a phrase which my Londoner colleagues and team-mates used on occasion. Though I couldn't quite bring myself to utter it, I liked its faint tinge of menace. A lady who was in the room that very evening later joined our staff at Saints.

'I was so frightened,' she confided in Ella. 'Is your husband bad-tempered?'

'Awful,' said my wife. 'You should have seen the Monkey God.'

XXI

Football in England was the breath and meaning of life. Once in Spain I had swum out from a remote shoreline to where a broken tower stood on a tiny island. Painted on the seaward side in white capitals was not 'My name is Ozymandias, King of Kings', but a briefer tag: 'Luton Town FC.' Football has a universality, or so I thought until arriving in Australia. Before our move the word soccer had never passed my lips, no more than it had the lips of 99% of the British population. The game was tentatively introduced at Saints by Mr Peter Wells in 1974. The general reaction was that the ebola virus had been released, or, put another way, that one's choice was between either the grandeur and manliness of Australian Rules football or Priscilla, Queen of the Desert. Elderly staff members' opinions generally began with, 'I never thought I would see the day...'

It took about six years of being patronised before a capable First Eleven walked out to play. It contained our son

Christopher who became one of four Roe generations of footballers, starting with my father, whose promising career was cut short by World War Two. Three Saints teams, 1982, 1988, and 1993 feared no schoolboy team in the country and after my retirement others emerged.

They generally played with a verve and will to attack and, just as importantly, with laughter not far away. One memorable event was the Great Shoe Mystery. We had just finished a hard-fought match to find, on returning to the changing-room, that everyone had lost a shoe, though only one, the other shoe remaining untouched. The culprit, an opposition player who had been sent off, eventually admitted, after a day's vehement denial facing the police, he had delivered the shoes to St Vincent de Paul's charity shop, an apparently pointless move, since who wants one shoe. The answer was that Vinnies had donated the shoes to the Amputees Association. Somehow we couldn't do the rounds asking for them back.

More and more capable players emerged and many wished to play together after leaving school. Soon our Old Scholars teams were also a force to be reckoned with, having to date won five major titles and a huge number of lesser ones, this despite being sea-green incorruptible amateurs where payments are concerned. Other clubs have expressed doubt about this and we have been labelled, particularly in the northern suburbs, as 'a drain on the tax-payers' purse', another of those delusions which somehow take on the air of a great truth. For a while we even acquired a ladies team, a paralogism that still mystifies me.

Adelaide's a city and all cities have at least a superficial resemblance, but no non-urban area that I know of resembles Australia, even superficially. The great Rockhampton trek was only scratching the surface. We more or less replicated it the next year by driving to Sydney and back, and school expeditions acquainted me with the Flinders Ranges, the fascinating Gammon Ranges, the Victorian Alps and the bleak south-west wilderness of

Tasmania. Then there was the Nullarbor expedition of 1978. This was a memorable adventure, involving nine boys, three adults and no fewer than eight camels. A coastal journey took us from Mundrabilla to Eucla along the Roe Plains, following the cliffs of the Bight with the sea immense below us, then turning inland to traverse as much of the Nullarbor as we could. We even ran a successful bird survey for the revised Australian Atlas of Birds which, to my surprise and gratification, included my name in its index. A couple of images: riding a camel over a red sandy terrain, the sea blue-grey to the right through occasional clumps of mulga trees, as Major Mitchell cockatoos, pink, white and orange floated almost tame among us: then in the central Nullarbor when, not riding, one walked seemingly always in a shallow saucer, unable ever to reach an illusory horizon, with endless permutations of stones or pebbles in every shade from rusty orange to a creamy white.

Years later Ella and I rode on The Ghan from Adelaide to Darwin, a four-day rail journey. She watched the interminable eucalypts without enthusiasm. 'It's all too empty for a girl from Walnut Place,' she said. In Kakadu we took a river cruise and saw crocodiles leap high from the water, emerging suddenly when meat was suspended on a line. At every leap she shrieked, enthralled by the power and strangeness of these prehistoric creatures.

In truth, her teenage joie de vivre, that had been almost extinguished by the drudgery and disillusionment of her first marriage, had returned in full. Australia had given her a confidence and a breadth of experience and acquaintance. These qualities appeared most clearly whenever she returned to England and was among her family and old friends. Her sisters-in-law, both of them strong-minded women, confided in me: 'She's a high-flyer,' said one.

'Once she got out of the cage,' said the other.

Twice we visited Moscow. These were the shut-down years of Brezhnev and Soviet paranoia. On our second visit she left her expensive and highly-esteemed suede coat on the plane.

'I think you've lost that,' I said spinelessly.

She was having none of this and strode off with two armed guards to restrain her. Some time passed. It was clearly necessary for me to find out to which Arctic labour camp she had been despatched. Sheremetyevo airport always seemed in a permanent twilight, but she emerged from the shadows still under guard, though wearing her coat. Apparently negotiating the release of the coat had been difficult since she and the customs officers were devoid of any mutual language.

'So what did you do?'

'The woman behind the desk was wearing my coat. But it was mine and I was having it.'

'I'm proud of you. Let's try the restaurant.'

'No thanks. Remember the last time?'

I remembered it well. On the previous visit we'd spent a week in Moscow. Despite our staying in the cobwebbed grandeur of the Metropole

Hotel the food was close to inedible, in Ella's case completely inedible, and after our first meal she had retired to bed, vomiting on the way. In a replica of her first pregnancy days she sent me out into the Soviet darkness to find food. Since Moscow had no version of Cleethorpes' Wonderland, choc-ices were nowhere to be found. In fact nothing was to be found except beetroots, until reaching the American embassy where a slot machine sold me a dozen Mars bars.

She recovered and we found our stay interesting, visiting the Kremlin, the Bolshoi Ballet and even taking a bus trip into the country-side. We did have a watcher who was a true patriot. When I had a coughing fit and blamed the brownish-yellow air, I was told Moscow air was the purest in the Soviet Union, which, if it was true, didn't say much for Stalingrad and the rest. We also visited the GUM department store, which was a stylish and impressive building, though completely empty of any merchandise. Our supervisor reassured us that a consignment of socks would arrive the next day, and if we were disappointed we could visit Lenin's Tomb. We declined on political grounds and also because the queue was four miles long.

'You'd have thought they had better things to do,' I surmised.

'Such as?' she said.

In 1991 came her favourite trip. We both had long service leave and thus the chance for a four-month holiday. Ella organised this entirely, thus meticulously. Our first destination was Zimbabwe, where we stayed with our friends the Kay family on their tobacco farm, visiting Peterhouse where pleasingly we had not been forgotten. Then, fulfilling an old promise, we saw Victoria Falls again, before visiting the Hwange Game Park, one of Africa's fine reservations. Here I wrote my name in the visitors' book and saw to my astonishment that had we been a week earlier we would have met my cousin Tom and his wife. Since he could barely walk, even with crutches, one could only admire his fortitude.

After England, and a fortnight with our parents, came our European venture, starting in Paris, then Limousin to stay with my sister in her remote farmhouse, then Florence and Venice. Staying in hotels or with friends we were more often than not provided with single beds, which meant when it came time to sleep my wife would complain of the cold and squeeze into my bed. This was nice enough, almost intoxicating in its own way, but crowded. Her solution was neat and easy.

'I'll stay here, now that it's nice and warm. You sleep in my bed.'

This exchange had a practicality about it hard to dispute and it extended across her personality. Her intellectual reactions reflected her mathematical mind-set. Things should behave in sequence and without dilettantism. In Paris at the Louvre she studied her catalogue as she looked at the pictures; in Florence she worked her way through the crowd until face to face with Michelangelo's 'David'; in Venice she visited Murano, the glassmaking island, and sat alongside a glass-maker so long that he eventually invited her to have a go, which was accepted at once.

She was fifty-seven years old at this time. Her hair was still red, her vigour unquenchable, and she loved life. I had in her someone who gave every day meaning. She energised my world. I believed she would never die, not in my awareness. The women rarely died first. Our own mothers outlived our fathers, as did Ella's sisters outlive their husbands; my brother's wife too became a widow as did my own sister. My two aunts and my great-aunt all lost their husbands and our four grandmothers were all widows, mine for sixteen and thirty-two years respectively.

Anyway it wasn't so much that she died that broke the pattern. It was the living death that came first, that took her so far away into a place I couldn't reach, a purgatory that made no sense.

Somehow not long before she died she remembered our days in Venice, almost paraphrasing Browning's lines:

... they lived once thus at Venice, where the merchants were the kings,
Where Saint Mark's is, where the Doges used to wed the sea with rings.

> *Ay, because the sea's the street
> there, and 'tis arched by ... what
> you call*
> *... Shylock's bridge with houses on
> it, where they kept the carnival...'*

From England our journey took us across the Atlantic to New Orleans, the home of her favoured jazz singers. The city was interesting and had its moments. As we strolled along Bourbon Street, Ella suggested having a drink in a bar, walked into one and came out immediately before I could follow, ushering me away.

'What's the matter?'

'There's a girl in there climbing a pole. You don't want to see it.'

Strip clubs always seemed sad places, so it didn't concern me a lot.

'OK,' I said. 'I'd sooner look at you anyway.'

'I'm not climbing any pole,' she said conclusively.

We booked a river trip on a Mississippi steam-boat. Neither of us had ever seen the river and when we climbed the levee its waters spread to the horizon like the sea. Ella in her excitement, burst into song, in fact into the original unsanitised lyrics, concerning African-Americans who 'all work on de Mississippi.'

I remember actually clapping my hand over her mouth. 'You'll get us lynched.'

There was a man on the levee, in a grubby white suit, playing a trumpet.

'I can play any tune in the world,' he said grandiloquently.

'All right. Play "The Road to Gundagai",' said Ella. He played it with masterful ease.

We crossed the Rockies by bus, stopping outside the Banff Springs Hotel. 'Only millionaires get off here,' shouted the driver and made to drive on.

'We're getting off,' said the girl from Walnut Place. It was an opulent hotel all right and a string quartet played waltzes far into the night. A new dress came out of one of her suitcases. She even got someone to iron it. I couldn't take my eyes off her and asked her for every dance.

Later back on our bus, I heard just behind me the familiar Lincolnshire accent. The man and I chatted: he was from Horncastle which was not far from Heighington. He knew my village.

'Know it well. I've a good friend who lives there. Harold Roe.'

'My father,' I said, resolving to re-read Arthur Koestler's *Roots of Coincidence*.

Our last visit was San Francisco. My memory of it is hazy, apart from one incident. The city has an abundance of trams and we were crossing a square when Ella's spiky heel got caught in a tramline. We struggled for some time to extricate it with no success until, inevitably, a tram appeared. It seemed unlikely to stop.

'Leave it,' I said.

'I'm certainly not leaving it! What do you mean "leave a shoe"! You can't be serious!'

With the rushing tram almost upon us she dragged the shoe out and sprang backwards, avoiding the tram with the sort of theatrical flourish that a matador uses evading an enraged bull.

Shoes have meant little to me. Usually I possess one pair of black shoes and one pair of brown suede. Then there are a couple of others of the sort of antique shabbiness that Harry White-Pallister approved of, friendly old shoes which Ella was inclined to throw away.

She was a shoe-lover and accumulator on an epic scale, or so it seemed to me. Even now her shoe-room houses forty-eight pairs, all seemingly new. I've just counted them. They're all boxed with neat labels such as 'Bronze, wear with tan suit'. There used to be more, lots more. Maybe forty-eight is par for the course for ladies, I'm not sure, but she could have had a thousand pairs had she so wished.

XXII

Our children were making their own way in the world. Christopher had flourished at St Peter's, as we had hoped. His final matriculation results were outstanding and more than justified our faith in his teachers. He went on to Adelaide University, eventually taking an Honours Degree in History which did not surprise me as he had been taught by Mr Fisher and Mr Roetman, confirming my fairly unoriginal belief that much of one's future depends on one's life intersecting with skilled mentors. It's chancy: they may have just retired, or taken a year off, or simply been time-tabled to a class not yours. Whatever will be will be.

Not everything went smoothly for him but, like our daughter, he found the right partner with whom to share life, thus winning the big lottery.

Our daughter, more than anyone else in our extended family of around fifty people, was likely to give the wheel a wrench if it behaved inequitably. She cantered through her school days first at East Adelaide and then at Saints Girls, as her secondary school seemed generally known.

All the school reports our children received are still in my possession and naturally we studied them carefully when they arrived. My favourite comment read: 'She has contributed vigorously in school sport'. This may have carried a whisper of irony in that Ella, going to watch a school hockey match, had arrived to find her daughter and a girl of the opposing team grappling on the grass like infuriated cats. My wife hauled them apart with words to the effect that she hadn't paid exorbitant school fees to watch guttersnipes fighting it out.

'A bit like your first morning at South Park,' I reminded her.

'That was different,' she said, though unable at once to pin-point the difference.

'As is the mother, so is the daughter,' I sought to remind her. 'Says so in the Bible. In Ezekiel.'

'Ezekiel! What does he know?' I thought it best to leave it there.

Madeleine went on to study Medicine at Flinders University and to come perilously close to being shown the door. After her first year examination she faced a number of supplementary examinations that broke a university record. There were tears and despondency but virtually the same thing had happened to me at Cambridge. This factor was used by Ella, arguing that knowing the experience would better fit me to provide a countermeasure. My instructions in remedial medicine were limited to saying: 'Let's learn it off by heart.' Sometimes it works. She passed the lot and the predicament never re-arose.

The mother-daughter relationship was not always clear. For instance, affairs of the heart were assessed by Ella and then the case referred to me, despite my protesting that it was 'secret women's business'. Eventually the problem solved itself when Madeleine returned from fifteen months in Antarctica to announce that she had a fiancé and her fiancé would ask my permission for him to become her fiancé. A prima facie case, until proved otherwise, which thus far shows no sign whatsoever of happening.

What was utterly clear was that mother and daughter loved and admired one another. Both had scientific and practical minds and when our daughter had qualified and gained experience in the medical profession she opted for a lengthy spell in Antarctica at Mawson Base. The utterly wretched years of her first marriage always rankled in Ella's mind. 'Cooped up with an habitual drunk in a house that stank of his vomit,' she said bitterly. 'A sexual relationship that lasted a few weeks, and that was too long. I knew little of the world other than the smell of beer. I'm nervous thinking of my daughter in that place of ice and whales, but it's a clean place, she's brave and she'll cope.'

She did better than cope. A life-saving feat of surgery saw her on the Queen's Honours List. The citation was glowing, including the sentence: 'Dr Madeleine Roe displayed great courage and extraordinary ability in the management of this remarkably difficult case.'

We were delighted and proud parents at the presentation ceremony at Government House in Adelaide. The champagne sparkled. The bitter cup was not close yet. One day we would both drink it empty.

The years rolled by, gradually increasing their speed of passage for some reason I've never been able to grasp, and 1995 saw me reach the age of sixty. For reasons we'll come to later I decided to retire from teaching.

So what did it all come down to, all those years in the cheerful company of my pupils and colleagues. It was as if it had passed in a flash, almost never happened at all, leaving me with a full quota of years and nowhere to go. Then the letters started to come in, almost a flood and, though the flow has long diminished, still the odd late-comer shows up, like a guest arriving at yesterday's party. What other profession would elicit them? Nurses? Doctors, perhaps? Maybe priests? The encomia, inflating my sense of worthiness and laudability ought realistically to have been punctured by an occasional communication to the effect that my lessons had been characterised by banality and the writer, even as a young boy, had found them shallow in content and tepid in delivery. In fact, I'm glad to say, there was no such letter, though there was one memorable phone-call from a lady making a similar deflating point on behalf of her son, concluding that she would further express her displeasure to the headmaster on the explicit grounds that she would rather deal with the organ-grinder than with the monkey.

One mother wrote that she enjoyed debating with her son, over the dinner-table, the contents of his day's lessons, but felt it unfair that the son saying, 'Mr Roe said...' was the indisputable conclusion to any discussion. There were so many who wrote and so grateful in content that they shall stay in their file, apart from two. The first was from a young man who was not above satirising me, even doing disrespectful though amusing impersonations, yet, years later, he took the trouble to write to me.

'You are truly one of the most interesting people I have met and known in my relatively short forty years. Thank you for helping so many boys like me visualise and live the dream.'

The second was the sort of letter one could only hope for and modesty forbids quoting the full content but the following words at least epitomised my aims, though their fulfilment was rarely mine to know.

'You taught me what it is to think, the importance of free thought and the beauty of communicating thought through language. Your lessons inspired me. I will always remember you.'

What does one say? Thank you, of course and one small but essential postscript: 'You just can't do it alone.'

Ella and I went to the musical *Chicago* at the Adelaide Festival Theatre. She loved the show and sang along with several of the lyrics. Her favourite, and she was fizzing with delight when the duet singing it (actually a trio when one added my wife) reached this final stanza:

Like the deserted bride on her
wedding night,
All alone and shaking with fright,

*With her brand new hubby nowhere
in sight:*
'I simply cannot do it alone'.

No-one can teach in a vacuum.
What's the point? The combination of
teacher and pupil isn't quite a symbiosis
but if it's operating as it should then
one could justifiably call it a fusion. No
teacher can do it alone.

At times, particularly in my younger
days, standing in front of a class
seemed strange.

'No, I am not Prince Hamlet nor was
meant to be:

Am an attendant lord, one that will
do

To swell a progress, start a scene
or two...'

Gradually I edged up the cast:
naturally it was Rozencrantz or
Guildenstern at first, then some loyal
unquestioning thane, such a one as
Ross in *Macbeth,* but eventually it would
have to be the lead. Being
imperturbably omniscient like Prospero,
or Mr Schubert, was out of my league.
No-one in Shakespeare seemed quite
to fit. Maybe a little less elevation?

Perhaps Biggles? Even when things were not quite under control he'd be backed up by Ginger and Algy: 'Cup o' cocoa, skipper?'

Biggles never married, though he did once have a brief romance with Marie, before she turned out to be a German spy. My luck held where Biggles' hopes collapsed, because I had Ella. At the interval of *Chicago* we had gone for a drink at the bar. As we worked our way through the crowd, heads turned. It was familiar enough. For occasions like this she would always dress up, put on what she called 'war-paint', and distract people with her good looks and vitality, leaving me the role of Mr Cellophane. The latter was one of my favourite songs in *Chicago*:

I tell ya, Cellophane, Mr
Cellophane, shoulda been my
name,
Mr Cellophane, 'cause you can look
right through me,
Walk right by me, never even
know I'm there...

Sometimes I would sing it at home, though she kindly disagreed on my transparency, even though we had both clearly heard a lady at the bar say, 'Who's the man with her?' and her companion respond: 'What man?'

What did it matter? Nothing wrong with being an unobtrusive but worthy person such as Atticus Finch in *To Kill a Mockingbird,* or since Atticus's wife was dead thus ruling him out, what about Dennis Thatcher who quietly played golf while his wife ran things.

We went to see *Evita,* in the year Ella retired. She pounced on the songs, not least 'Don't cry for me Argentina'.

It won't be easy, you'll think it's strange
When I try to explain how I feel,
That I still need your love after all that I've done,
You won't believe me, all you will see is a girl you once knew
Although she's dressed up to the nines ...

Ella was singing her own life, we both knew.

I had to let it happen, I had to change

*Couldn't stay all my life down at
heel
Looking out of the windows,
staying out of the sun,
So I chose freedom ...*

To be honest being arm-in-arm with
her was really nothing like being Mr
Cellophane. If anything it was like being
the man who broke the bank at Monte
Carlo.

XXIII

Saints for almost all my tenure there kindly allocated me the top Year Eleven set, they thus boasting the title 11JR. Invariably they were a delight to teach. It wasn't work at all, it was just absorbing fun. There was no phantom authority to suggest one should really teach this or that. In so far as there was a target it was with us, and I'm sure among my colleagues teaching the humanities, to encourage a diversity of thought and to try to provide the stimuli that would help this to happen. We read widely: Conrad, Lawrence, Orwell, Solzhenitsyn, and the Bronte sisters, among a variety of others, tossing Beckett, Pinter and Kafka into the mix, plus Steinbeck, Greene and Fitzgerald. The school uncomplainingly came up with my requests for the texts.

We worked on the ease of expression, on varieties of tone, we forebade stereotypes, unless satirising them. Their poetry was a joy to read, often drawn to the iambic pentameter as a rhythm and thus the sonnet as a

form. The notion of the poetic image
and the tension between intellect and
imagination seemed to fascinate. There
were lively controversies, one that sticks
in my mind being whether or not
beauty lies in the eye of the beholder,
a question that usually caused a
vigorous fifty-fifty split in the class.
Another focus was the function of the
word. Can one think without words? In
no time we worked out that one can't,
other than as a sort of primal jelly-fish
response. The class jumped all over
1984: Big Brother wants fewer words.
Which word does he most want to
eliminate? 'Freedom,' they said. 'No
place for that in Newspeak, unless you
make it mean slavery.'

Rarely did a lesson pass without
merriment, the boys even cheerfully
analysing laughter as a phenomenon.
There were memorable moments: we
were considering (don't ask me why)
what single question would one ask
God, should the opportunity arise. There
was some conventionality, e.g. 'Is there
an after-life, God?' but what became by
acclaim 'the people's question' was
whether the toy building blocks, i.e.

Lego, were pronounced 'Leggo' or 'Laygo'.

Sometimes I liked to sit in a vacant desk among my pupils and do some writing myself, listening for that sussuration that said the hive was thinking. The hive and I once wrote Country and Western lyrics but they were so melancholy it put me off C&W for some time.

I live back in the woods, you see,
My woman, my kids, my dog and
me ...

OK so far, until Billy-Joe McCafferty shot their dog.

Ella enjoyed discussing classroom technique and ethics, she being now teaching full-time and very successfully. She liked to hear about my one junior class who were probably like junior classes the world over and could not believe their teachers existed outside the classroom. So they took it as fiction when I told them of two Lancaster bombers falling simultaneously from the blackness, landing not far from our family house, their bomb-loads exploding with a deafening roar and a glaring intensity, the blast tearing our back door and two inner doors off their hinges. That night will never leave the eight-year-old boy that I was.

My one history class was enjoyable too, particularly as it dealt with Medieval European history, a period that for most was tabula rasa, which led us down the blindest of alleys at times. For instance, we were discussing the historical roles of various animals, easy and interesting in the case, say, of the ox or camel, but more abstruse when a pupil asked what was the historical contribution of the wombat. Doing my best to be scholarly I surmised that they had been a source of meat, though being sorely tempted to describe the giant wooden wombat that had played so significant a part in the siege of Troy. Of course, there were endless opportunities for contention: for instance, whether Magellan's starving crew in mid-Pacific were really reduced, according to reputable historians, to eating the leather casings of their ship's mast. This was disputed vehemently ('Impossible. Couldn't be done.') So we agreed that if the most rigorous denier could eat his own leather belt then Form 9RF would accept Magellan's chroniclers' words. We marinated chopped up parts of the boy's belt for a fortnight or so and he nobly proved himself wrong by eating a portion of it.

English and History classes alike need a hard core and proper preparation but diversion was never far away, though I usually preferred it towards the lesson's end, or we'd never have done anything. Once we were considering whether a monkey, given infinite time, could type out the entire works of Shakespeare. Small boys don't like infinity.

'Sir, how much would the monkey have typed out by the end of next week?'

Being unable to say one could only hazard a guess. 'Well, if it's typed out 'G.o.o.d' then it's made a start on *Timon of Athens*.'

'Never heard of it.'

'Well, Pocklington, the monkey's probably never heard of it either. But he's given it his best shot. An example for all of us, I think.'

A boy in one junior class gave me a copy of *Noddy Meets the Elves.* Noddy was my lowest-ranking rung in the literary ladder but from time to time it was hard to resist reading aloud from it. A few lines on Noddy picking flowers, then both tone and plot changed. 'The giant anaconda slithered through the flowers, coiled around Noddy and crushed the poor little fellow to death, before...'

'Sir, that's not true! Is it?'

'No, it isn't. It was in fact a giant boa constrictor.'

I suppose we got the details right eventually.

Somehow or other the younger boys were never downhearted despite regularly protesting that they were overworked. Once, wanting to see how they handled a fairly abstract topic, I proposed they should write on the subject of time. This was almost the first lesson of the year and therefore, they informed me, their essay should rather be on what they had done in their holidays, on the grounds that this time-honoured title had been set every year since they were four.

'But I already know,' I said. 'You played cricket in the backyard and went to your, or someone else's, beach-house. Apart from the boarders, of course, who have to go off and mend the rabbit-proof fence.'

Trying to explain Platonic ideals to my matriculation class I liked to use this holiday as an example of the true ideal of which every other holiday is only a dim reflection.

My matriculation class was different, since for them the results of their final examination could well make a significant difference to their futures. So we worked seriously (some of the time). There were surprises for me as one of my rules was to pick fairly demanding literature, preferring Dickens, Lawrence and, among the poets, Gerard Manley Hopkins. It took me a year or two to realise that Australia had produced a great and moving novelist in Patrick White. He should be compulsory reading the world over.

Whether there was a common thread that ran through it all is uncertain, but one of my colleagues once told me my teaching technique could be abbreviated thus:

If you want flotsam, I've got some,
If you want jetsam, I can get
some.

To this day I haven't decided whether it was a compliment or not. About sixty–forty not, at a guess.

December 1995 saw my retirement. The reasons for this are not altogether clear to me even now, other than a suspicion that there were signs of self-parody in my teaching, which if so would have been regrettable. To respect our professions was always, both for Ella and me, the over-riding criterion. It was no secret that as head of her department she had given one instructor a scathing dressing-down, on the lines of his being there to teach, not to use his position for his own interests.

However, there was another reason for my farewell to my friends, pupils and colleagues alike. George Bernard Shaw, in *Man and Superman* produces the line: 'He who can does, he who cannot teaches.' Shaw did not add, as was not uncommon in staff rooms, 'He who cannot teach, teaches teachers.' But Shaw's aphorism niggled me. Years of explaining the art and design of the novel, yet never having written one, nor seriously attempted such a project, seemed not quite satisfactory.

So throughout 1996 much of my attention was concentrated upon writing something that might possibly develop into a novel. Ella was still teaching, thus most of the day, apart from holidays, was spent alone. A book that has for years fascinated me is Teilhard de Chardin's *The Phenomenon of Man.* Even now it is kept permanently by my bedside as a sort of gymnasium for my mind. His central hypothesis is that the universe is always in a state of flux, striving towards and becoming new levels of existence: insofar as one can put it in a phrase, 'the inevitable necessity of evolution'. Since mankind is, on our planet at least, the spearhead of this process, de Chardin analyses where evolution will, and has to, take us.

This so interested me that my attempt at a novel dealt, for better or worse, with what seemed to me a possible early evolutionary development, this being set in a relatively near future. Pre-eminently a novel tells a story, thus needing a plot and characters who move or are moved around by the central proposition. The process of writing was fascinating in that the novel began to resemble an organism. I'm not sure if this is a commonly recognised quality, but the story almost functioned on its own. In the final third of the tale the characters' actions and speech seemed not mine but their own, almost a form of dictation.

Gradually, though it was completely unintentional, the central female character, Kit, came to resemble Ella, not, of course, identically but in several ways. Kit had red hair and was stubborn and determined. Her falling in love has set-backs. She is slightly deformed, which Ella was not. In my earliest teaching days, one of my pupils, 'Little Jim' Wetherald, had a hand so deformed it was almost a paw. He always wore a black glove. It was as well to make no comment on this as his classmates were ferociously supportive of him. Jim was tenacious and tough and I admired him. I wanted his spirit in the story, not least because my wife shared it.

My composing the story was done entirely in pen and ink, but Ella watched over the process and every ten pages or so would type it into her computer. She made occasional suggestions and once wrote a brief passage herself. 'To her Jacky seemed to stroll through the world, not noticing its menaces and pitfalls, and to her half-amused impatience it seemed as if the world sympathised with him, rather as if it would be on its best behaviour because that was how he expected it to be.'

'That's you,' she said. 'Born lucky.'

I liked the passage and it fitted the character though Jacky was not the person through whom I was moving the central ideas. At the time it seemed a comforting verdict which goes to show how sardonic fate can be. 'Wyn eal gedreas', said the Saxons. 'All the joy has died'. Or would before long, and our world wouldn't be on its best behaviour or hospitable or generous at all. I'm not so sure about 'lucky' either.

Ella was happy in her work at TAFE in the Fashion and Design department. She was occasionally at cross-purposes with the management, but after a while became head of the faculty. It provided, reputedly, the best course of its type in Australia and demand for places was always high. There were regular fashion shows, not only the end of year parades but interstate jaunts to Sydney and Melbourne. Among several Sydney exhibitions was one which she described as 'pretty unorthodox', this taking place in Redfern in what was, according to her, a cavernous warehouse.

Knowing her they would be organised and high quality, and probably good fun as her team demonstrated at St Peter's College when she was persuaded to run a fashion show as part of a fundraiser for a cricket tour. This went well from the start and a largely male audience, judging by the applause, were further delighted when the girls modelling dresses switched to parading in bikinis.

The department was large and she dealt capably, as one would expect, with its finances. Her fairness in allocating funds made her highly regarded in departments such as the carpenters and electricians. The younger trades apprentices sometimes gathered their chairs at coffee time under a metal spiral staircase leading down from the fashion area, thus enabling them to ogle the ladies climbing or descending. It took a good deal more than this to daunt my wife's confidence; once having unconcernedly gone up the steps, she turned and called down: 'If you see anything new you will tell me, won't you?'

She cared for those she worked with, pupils and colleagues alike: for instance she provided special food for visiting Malaysian students, identified and helped drug-dependent students, or ones who were potentially suicidal, or single mothers with young children. The previous head of her faculty had crossed swords with Ella from time to time, but when this lady developed motor neurone disease my wife would drive her to her hospital appointments, often waiting hours while treatment took place. She even analysed pension schemes for her fellow-instructors, working through the small print to select the most lucrative.

About a year after her death I saw her for a moment in Norwood, our closest large suburb, walking on the other side of the road. Her red hair was unmistakable, before she disappeared into a shopping mall. I called out, 'Ella, wait!' and began to run, stopping after a dozen paces as reality restored its pointless familiar greyness. A few shoppers glanced half-curiously.

The delusion would in itself hardly merit any mention except that it mirrored thousands of previous moments. After Ella died the stark truth came that never again would there be that uplifting energising moment when she came into sight. From the first day we met until the long dreadful vigil on the day she died there had always been this almost galvanic response. Twice she went to England on her own and I had awaited her return in the airport reception area, staring at the plane as it landed and then at the passengers emerging from the customs transit, fretting lest she be delayed, wondering why so many anonymous people were taking precedence. Then she appeared and I would find myself pushing forward and waving. In their own way these were extreme cases and plenty of other people alongside me were equally likely to be waiting anxiously and expectantly. But the same recognition process happened on the most everyday occasions. Sometimes she would come to watch my football games and I was uneasy until establishing where she was placed among other spectators, repeating exactly the same ritual when I was batting or fielding at cricket. It has fallen to me to give a good many speeches, some with disastrous consequences, of which more later, but always they went well provided she was present and in clear view. She was my talisman, elemental and lucky: I couldn't lose. No doubt this sounds self-indulgently sentimental and mawkish, but so be it. If you'd known her you would have understood. Anyway this is a love story.

Our first grandson, Robert Harold, was born in the last month of Ella's employment at TAFE. She promptly retired from work. A few years later another grandson, Alexander Marcus, was born, both being the children of Christopher and his wife Kristin. We saw the boys often and did our best to make their childhood days memorable and entertaining. There was an electric train set, miniature cars, toy soldiers, jigsaws, playing-cards, and, naturally, the resurrected figures of Rupert and Rumpelstiltskin. Outside was the pool, with a boat and a large crocodile, both inflated and perfect for the exploits of Tarzan. They've been stored away now, crocodile and toys alike.

Dragons live for ever, but not so little boys,
Little Jackie Paper has put away his toys.

Both had inherited sporting genes, were good soccer players and talented cricketers. Their grandmother watched over them and loved it when they stayed overnight. Backyard cricket went on for hour after hour under rigorous rules. Once a memorable moment occurred when a ball was hit towards mid-on, where it passed close to a large Eastern Brown, a snake reckoned the world's second most venomous land-snake, more deadly even than the notorious Nag the Cobra. There were cries of: 'Look at that snake! Where's it supposed to be fielding?' A technical debate followed, pondering why the snake was too far back from the batsman to stop any single, but not far enough back to prevent a boundary. 'What's your captain thinking, snake?' said our eight-year-old grandson in disgust. It could only happen in Australia. Nearer their home the boys would practise in the local park's nets, on worn dusty matting, the iron stumps chained to the rusted aviary-like enclosure of the wire netting, in temperatures always seemingly 38°C, sweat dripping off their faces, two young lads dressed in scruffy T-shirts and shorts though fully gloved and padded, batting on. It must have been something like that for the children of Sparta.

One wondered at times what their mother, with her German background, made of it all. She did occasionally protest at family dinners that the company might consider a conversation other than on cricket, which produced a truce lasting about ninety seconds.

If the boys ever look back on those wonderful days when grandma Ella put Band-Aids on their cuts and sun-screen on their faces, cooked their favourite roast potatoes and made her much-admired trifles, when she emerged to forbid bowling bouncers at little Alex (particularly when he dispatched one through her stained-glass window), do they remember her as she was then or, as hospital visitors, do they remember the poor broken soul of her last years.

I remember a lot of the good times and the bad, though not everything. Yesterday as I drove home I heard someone singing on the car radio. The few words I caught were not from any song I'd ever heard, but they made me tremble and sob:

It all fades away, but you,
It all fades away, it all fades away,
It all fades away, but you.

Those years after we retired and before our little world collapsed, a dozen or so of years, I suppose, seem, looking back, a golden time, hazy in my memory but shining as soap-bubbles shine. In my Essex days I had several times stood in the crowd at West Ham United's grand old stadium, Boleyn Ground. (Ann Boleyn, Henry VIII's second wife, supposedly had lived adjacent). Whenever I heard West Ham supporters in the crowd sing their special song it was oddly touching:

I'm forever blowing bubbles,
Pretty bubbles in the air,
They fly so high, nearly reach the sky,
Then like our dreams, they fade and die.

Our dreams, Ella's and mine, had flown high and nearly reached the sky. So what's left to tell now is the dreams' deaths.

For some reason or other I found myself delivering at least two or three lectures per year. This was always entertaining and made me do some serious research. The Literary Society were kind enough to ask me once a year; there were lectures at the Adelaide State Library and the Matthew Flinders Society among others, as well as various St Peter's functions. The topics were whatever caught my fancy: 'Speaking Anglo-Saxon', 'Jane Austen's family', 'The men who wrote the King James Bible', 'Imperial Literature', 'Kipling's childhood', 'The education of Elizabeth I' and 'A Lincolnshire village'. This was the tiny village of Donington, with which I was familiar, and had within twenty years produced two remarkable contemporaries, Joseph Banks and Matthew Flinders.

There were unexpected moments. Twice the Literary Society was unable to find a venue other than a restaurant, not telling me this until I arrived. On one occasion there were only a few patrons in the restaurant, as opposed to members of the society, and it was possible to involve them in the topic, which they seemed to enjoy, as no-one threw a bread roll at me. The second time was trickier, being in a packed and noisy Italian restaurant, where the Society's regulars and the cheerful talkative family groups simultaneously learned about Princess Elizabeth Tudor's education. Such a speech really needed the oratory of Marcus Tullius Cicero himself. Not possessing this I fell back on a series of invitations for the audience as a whole to fill their glasses and drink with me to the young princess, to her mother Ann Boleyn, to Titian the great Italian artist of that time, to the unfairly maligned Borgia family, and, to rapturous applause, to the Azzurri, Italy's football team which had just won the World Cup, this being 2006. Normally during these lectures I would try to catch Ella's eye so that she could signal her approval, or lack of it. This time it was equivocal as she was laughing hysterically while also gesturing 'thumbs down'.

However the lectures themselves were, in the long run, insignificant, relative to the totally unforeseen and unforeseeable impact of the Literary Society's secretary. She was a most pleasant and helpful lady who ran the Society enthusiastically and well. Her name was Gina, which I'm unlikely to forget having heard it thousands of times, it eventually having the same effect on my psyche as the name Stalingrad reputedly had upon Hitler.

Our retirement did seem for some years to be the happy companionship we had hoped for and, I think, expected. As I write I can glance around the room and see four intricately woven framed tapestries on the wall, including one of a unicorn done in white silk stitches so minute that one has to get very close to see that they actually exist. Ella loved tapestry and now having the time produced creations I could only marvel at. We continued to travel, going to England, Hong Kong and, in Australia, Darwin, Cairns (belatedly reaching the Barrier Reef) and several times to Tasmania where our daughter and her husband resided.

As Ella reached her seventies her health began to deteriorate. She had two knee replacements, high blood pressure and was taking what seemed an inordinate amount of medication. With her lack of physical activity her weight began to increase rapidly. Considering my daughter and daughter-in-law are both doctors my own knowledge of medicine is close to zero. My general good health no doubt has contributed to my fortunate unfamiliarity with illness. All my injuries have been sporting ones and to this day my intake of tablets or any medication apart from eye-drops or an occasional aspirin for tooth-ache has been and is nil.

So medical terms tend to mean nothing. Recently someone mentioned Asperger's Syndrome. It meant nothing. It was just a couple of words. What it affected was a mystery. It could have been hair loss or arthritis. So it was with dementia, even more so with Alzheimer's Disease. Now you know the name of the demon. Let me tell you about it. I have to, you see, though I'd sooner tell you about Dachau or Belsen or Auschwitz.

Alois Alzheimer was born in 1864 and in 1906 discovered and noted the characteristic plaques and tangles, which look like black stains, on the brain cells. They are rogue proteins which affect and eventually destroy the neurons which enable memory to exist. By the mid-century this disease is predicted to become mankind's second most lethal killer, after heart disease. It is eventually fatal in that the enfeebled mind simply loses its memory of how to live, or how the body operates. In the years before death the disease erodes the memory, gradually taking away one's remembered life, one's recalled autobiography. Eventually, strangers to themselves, one's loved ones slide into an inescapable abyss, a fate which awaits, should there be no cure, one in three human beings born in the decade after 2010.

With our longer lives Alzheimer's Disease is so ever-present that most of us know a sufferer, particularly if it is a family member. In the distant past it was probably designated as madness or possession or just the forgetfulness of old age. There was a period when Freud's psychotherapy tried to analyse the condition, but there was no need for id, ego, super-ego and so on. Alzheimer told us correctly it was a biological and cellular problem. We know now the actual malfunctioning protein that causes plaques to appear. It is amyloid. But though we know it affects memory, what we don't know is what memory is. In *Mansfield Park* Jane Austen wrote, 'If any faculty of our nature may be called more wonderful than the rest, I do think it is memory.' We know that short-term memory is the first to go, as indeed it was with Ella.

Probably humanity will find a way to defeat Alzheimer's but not before it is a global pandemic. As life expectancy increases so will the disease. Yet a decade ago it meant nothing whatever to me. I was truthfully ignorant of it, and so probably were most Germans ignorant of the holocaust.

My cousins Barbara and Alfred Curtis, my close friend Barbara Graham, my irrepressibly vivacious friend Judy Abbott, all shared two things. They were strong and talented personalities, distinct, unique, having lived full lives, but they could not have imagined, in their prime, what awaited them, no more than could Margaret Thatcher or Ronald Reagan. Alzheimer's knows no mercy. When in my dreadful nightmares, in the palatial antiques building, I fought the demon, I knew it meant to show me no mercy. Perhaps, possibly, probably we'll meet again one day, and it will take away my memory and the memories of Ella that I carry. That's really why I'm writing this. Lest I forget.

XXIV

For Ella's seventieth birthday we went to England. Our visit coincided with her younger brother, David, having his sixtieth birthday. At the big family gathering she was as bouncy and high-spirited as ever. They were happy times, relaxed and leisurely as retirement ought to be. The next year my wife organised, almost without my knowledge, a large and lively party for my seventieth birthday. My eightieth was in a year so utterly desperate, culminating in Ella's death, that had its melancholy progress been foretold it would have met, I'm certain, with disbelief. Getting old was an autumnal journey but so far enjoyable. Both our mothers had died in 1995, alert, lively and self-sufficient to the end. Wasn't that how it was supposed to be?

The dreadful future was first to clothe itself in reality in 2010. It was so appalling in its horrible strangeness that my mind has never properly encompassed it. Try as I will to remember, there are two or three years that seem to have, in large part, obliterated themselves, or merged with adjacent years. The demon was loose, and its power was overwhelming. In its shadow nothing made any sense. How can it be that, however hard one tries, there is no sequence, no order, no logic, by which to regulate those empty times. It was as if my brain was paralysed.

Somewhere, sometime, there must have been a finality to Ella's normal life. The last grain of sand must have fallen through the hourglass, there must have been a first struggle with the demon in its huge glass exhibition building. There were clues, I'm sure, though probably most passed me by, or I rationalised them as being part of the inevitable infirmity of old age: the more elderly, the more forgetful, the more prone to accidents. Nothing strange about that.

A photograph of Ella in a restaurant might have been an early hint. It looks normal enough to most people, I suppose, but it wasn't. She was fastidious about her appearance, in private and in public always smartly dressed, but the picture shows her hair untidy and she has no make-up. Then came more overt signals. There was the incident when she could not cope with the details of our financial affairs. It saddened and shook me that such an all-embracing skill-set should vanish so suddenly.

Then came another incident. We were having lunch at my golf club, a fairly formal affair with the chef carving roast meat and so on. I collected my plate from him and glanced around to find Ella. She was standing perfectly still, among the tables, holding her plate. She had filled it to overflowing with tomato soup, immersing the meat and vegetables. There were people staring. 'Never mind. It doesn't matter. It's all right. I'll get you another plate.' The chef replaced the meal swiftly and that was that, other than the scene lingering like a lesion in my mind.

As far as possible it required me to watch carefully over her, but this was nothing new, and for that matter she used to watch over and care for me. Then came a disturbing incident at home. An unfamiliar brightness caused me to look up towards the kitchen, where there were flickering shadows. Dashing there I saw Ella standing close to a column of fire, a metre high, that was coming from a saucepan of cooking fat. Flinging a towel over the pan I snatched it up, dashed outside, and hurled its contents into a flower-bed. Fortunately that dealt with the crisis. But she never cooked again. Not once.

She had been such an accomplished cook. There seemed no dish she could not serve up from her library of cooking manuals. Her pastries were a special delight and her trifles so mouth-watering that little Alex would open the fridge simply to gaze on the many-coloured delicacy. On the day the football season ended my teammates would gather at our house. 'Will she do curry again? For twenty of us?' She did, to everyone's approval. Christmas lunch was her master-piece. Sumptuous course after course emerged from the kitchen to be consumed with gusto by a table full of guests, after which she would retire to bed saying, 'That's enough for me. Somebody else can clear up.'

Gradually other skills shredded away. She had always been an excellent car-driver and actually understood the mechanism of cars, unlike my own approach which was to hope the car bonnet remained permanently closed. She began to get lost, or at least delayed, until the day that she was so late that I rang the police. They did their stuff and found her but it was clear that she could not find her way home. Driving now being out of the question for her, it became necessary for me to drive wherever she wished to go. This was no hardship, but what became clear was that I must not leave her alone. On one occasion thoughtlessly I got out of the car confident that it would take only a couple of minutes and that it was, anyway, raining so heavily it would surely deter her from leaving the car. My heart sank on returning to find she had gone. After what seemed an age of frustration and anxiety patrolling the streets, relief came when a kindly lady emerged from a shop to say Ella was sheltering inside.

These misadventures were stressful enough but somehow they felt manageable. It meant caring for her almost as one might with a child, but surely that was what marriage meant. Also I knew with total certainty that, had our circumstances been reversed, she would have been a loving and devoted guardian. Though now something of dementia is known to me, that was not the case at the time. Anyway she was my heart's delight, how could she possibly be demented. My mind revulsed at and rejected the very word. And the word 'madness'! My wonderful girl 'mad'? It could never be. It was some aberration that time and perhaps medication would resolve. This was the twenty-first century, wasn't it? Surely there weren't still demons?

So far, though saddening, the predicament demanded, or so it seemed then, patience and gentleness. What was to come was far, far worse. When the real torment actually began isn't possible to say, but there obviously must have been a first time when the cruel accusation was spoken. It would presumably have been engendered in her mind before it was spoken. The hateful, hopeless unreality of it was what made me wonder if this was more than mere amnesia.

Earlier I mentioned Gina, the Literary Society's secretary. She was lively and personable and to be perfectly accurate her real self plays no part in this story, other than inviting me once a year to deliver a talk to the Society. Her depressing and imaginary role was to be a sick image that had somehow entered Ella's mind. At some dark moment in, I'm fairly sure, 2010, my wife first accused me of infidelity. It was both morbid and inexplicably weird, but most of all it struck centrally and destructively at the single most deeply-held value of my entire life. I loved Ella. It was a simple and unvarying truth.

The accusation so offended me that I refused ever to countenance it, and whenever it was made, and it could be multiple times in any one day or night, would deny it utterly. A psychiatrist who helped us later on suggested that a more placatory response might help, but it was beyond me ever to appease this lie. It wasn't actually a lie, I suppose, though it certainly was both a falsehood and a wretched demeaning chimera.

It brought with it an elaborate fantasy so explicit that my mind felt almost delirious when the ritual interrogations were taking place. As closely as the phantasmagoria can be reproduced, here is some of what was repeated closely day after day, night after night, wracking our minds and wrecking our health.

'Have you seen your whore, Gina, today?'

'She's not a whore. She's a nice decent lady.'

'Then why are you sleeping with her?'

'I'm not. Don't say that.'

'I will say it, because it's true.'

'It's not true. It's nonsense.'

'Well, you're bound to say that. Anyway where were you all last night?'

'Here in bed, asleep, with you.'

'No, you weren't. I heard the car go out.'

'You couldn't. I was here.'

'You were at her house.'

'Please don't go on with this.'

'I saw you at her house.'

'No, you didn't. I don't even know where her house is.'

This was true enough and still is, but to demonstrate how the inquisitions affected me, I actually found scissors and cut the lady's name and address out of our telephone directory, while deliberately avoiding looking closely at the page, in order truthfully to deny knowing where she lived.

'Of course you know where it is. It's in Hatswell Street.'

'I'm sure it isn't.'

'Well, why are you always parking on Hatswell Street?'

'Because it's adjacent to St Peter's College and about ten yards away from the playing fields.'

'About ten yards from her house.'

'Why don't you ask the players? They'll tell you where I was.'

'They'll say anything you tell them.'

'Well, next time come with me.'

'Why don't you love me anymore?'

'I've always loved you. Always. You must know that.'

'Then why do you keep seeing your whore?'

'She's not a whore. You've got it all wrong.'

'I know you're seeing her.'

'I'm not.'

'Then why were you in her house the other night?'

'I can't go on with this.'

'Admit you're having an affair.'

'I'm not. I'm not. I'm not. I'm not.'

'Madeleine saw you going into her house.'

'Madeleine's in Tasmania.'

'She saw you when she was last here.'

'No, she didn't.'

'Chris saw you too. All three of us saw you. We followed you into her house.'

'How could you? I don't even know where it is.'

'It's on Hatswell Street.'

Like some insidious brain-washing it went on and on, literally hour after hour, day after day. Once, in sheer desperation, I persuaded her to go to Hatswell Street and visit the house in question. The street is short, has relatively few houses, as well as a factory, a playing-field and some warehouses. She pointed at a house.

'Let's go in and ask for Gina,' I said.

She refused. I knocked and an elderly lady carrying a hearing-aid opened the door.

'Does Gina live here?' Every instinct told me to disengage: even standing there was a sort of compliance in the whole sick fantasy.

'Have you brought the batteries?' said the lady.

'No, I haven't. Does Gina live here?'

'Zena?'

'I'm sorry I bothered you.'

Thinking that it's not only history that repeats itself first as tragedy then as farce, I returned to the car.

'If that's the house you mean, you are sadly mistaken.'

'When I went in there last night you were sitting on a stool near the fire. There isn't any doubt about it. She was there. There was a fat woman as well. Are you having an affair with her too?'

Once I would have said, 'That must have been Zena,' but those days had gone.

XXV

You may wonder at my forlorn hope that things might one day get better, but I knew nothing whatever of Alzheimer's Disease, in fact nothing of mental illness at all. Somehow there was still hope. We can see this through. The wheel will turn, provided we stick together.

Playing sport, particularly as captain or coach, with our team under desperate pressure, my policy was always to hang on: just stay in the game, our turn will come. Naively I wanted it to be true with her illness. But it turned out not to be a game at all, just anguish that almost sent me insane and, far worse, was to cost my love her life.

For about eighteen months this private struggle went on. Each day was like the one before, a calendar of repetitive abuse. It would grow worse when night came, apparently a common phenomenon of mental illness, known as the 'sundowner effect'. As we lay in bed I would try to hold her hand but nothing stemmed the questioning.

'Have you seen your whore today?'

'I don't know what you mean.'

'When did you last see Gina?'

'At a Literary Society lecture, nearly two years ago.'

'Why are you lying?'

'I'm not lying.'

Literally there were hundreds of nights like this and usually it meant my going into another bedroom. Then after a few minutes the door would open, the light be switched on and she was standing in the doorway.

'Please go to sleep,' I would mutter, eyes hurting from the sudden light.

'If I do you'll go over to her house.'

This sequence would take place repeatedly, often as many as ten times per night. Sometimes I would take refuge by sitting in the car for a few minutes of darkness in the garage, knowing that when this brief respite was over there would be allegations of having driven to Hatswell Street and back.

Lest this all sound, as indeed it does, an exercise in self-pity, what did not escape me was knowing that while my life was miserable how much worse was hers, bitter in having, as she thought, her love rejected and paltry. Paradoxically she mattered more than ever in her vulnerability.

The plight we were both in showed itself in other ways. I once stepped casually onto the bathroom scales, looked down and assumed they were broken. Stepping off and on again didn't work. The dial still showed 140lbs (or 63kg to you) so obviously it was faulty. My weight had varied very little since I was about thirty years old, always the same 178lbs (81kg). Clearly we needed new scales. The next day I noticed a weighing machine in the post office and stood on it. 63kg. More than a fifth of my body-weight had gone, vanished without my noticing, a psychosomatic disorder if ever there was one.

Another similar reaction also made its spasmodic presence felt about this time. This was a sudden and completely unpredictable vomiting. It went further than simply being sick; there was so much vomit it was hard to believe, but what appalled me far more than the volume was the unpredictability. The retching and convulsion came without even the slightest warning. For instance, while shopping in a large gardening store, I found myself kneeling on the floor, helpless to stop my stomach's convulsions. By good fortune no-one saw this humiliation, thanks to my being hidden by sacks of lawn seed in an out-of-the-way part of the store. Shamefacedly leaving a pool of vomit I got up and walked away. Another gross, self-inflicted indignity was vomiting while driving. Again it came utterly without warning, again a grotesque volume of semi-digested liquefaction, only this time soaking my shirt and trousers. Somehow I got the car out of the busy traffic. There were several similar incidents, so mortifying they are best forgotten.

After my infant school education I had progressed to a very tough elementary school of pupils aged from seven to fifteen. One commandment might appropriately have been sculpted in stone over its entrance: 'Boys do not cry'. There were some hard cases there, boys and staff, who could dish it out, but one choked back the tears. Nor were there tears for over seventy years, partly because life was generally happy, partly because of the ingrained code. Looking after Ella took almost every moment of my life in the years 2010 and 2011 and playing golf just about disappeared. Once, however, a kindly neighbour volunteered to keep Ella company while I played. In one of those frozen memories that my mind chooses to accumulate, the scene is as if it were happening now. On the front edge of the third green at Mount Osmond Golf Club my body refused to go on. I stood there, holding a putter, and began to weep. My playing group drew near and stood amazed. The thought came to me that this was how suicides must feel: what is the point of going on? Probably it was short-lived, as it was contrary to my own ethos, however childish, to 'stay in the game'. Ian and Paul, my partners, saw the tears and, though knowing nothing of my circumstances, were perceptive and quick to act. They escorted me off the course and back home, Ian driving my car and Paul following in his. I hope they eventually finished their round. From then on my acquaintance with tears has been frequent. In a way they seem to help.

And what are you that missing you,
I should be kept awake
As many nights as there are days
With weeping for your sake.

They were dreadful times. Only on November 29th, 2011 did I even hear the words 'Alzheimer's Disease' spoken. My responses to Ella's illness were two-fold and, I suppose, irresponsibly amateurish. Firstly was my denial that she was 'demented' or 'mad'. The very words appalled me. How could it be possible with her clear all-embracing intelligence. It seemed inconceivable and insulting to her. This led to my second knee-jerk of a reaction, which was to get more protective still. This was my wife and my beloved. It had fallen to me to care for her. There seemed to be no problem other than my supposed infidelity. This obsession was so utterly devoid of any evidence or credibility that time and common sense would surely cause it to vanish. There were various other areas, for instance my lack of interest in financial affairs, which could be seen as irresponsible or culpable, yet here she was utterly bedevilled with this imaginary affair. There only seemed to be the one, other than a stray reference or two to the unlikely 'fat woman' of Hatswell Street. I had always loved Ella passionately and she had always reciprocated, knowing and rejoicing that this was so. It was the treasured high-point of my life, irreproachable and fulfilling, belonging to another and better world than this squalid talk of whores and affairs.

Then events began to accelerate. Our daughter Madeleine returned from her third spell in Antarctica and kindly volunteered to care for her mother while I went to England for three weeks to watch our grandson Robert playing cricket there. It seemed a good idea at the time, my daughter being skilled in medicine and being very close to her mother. Also I would return refreshed, or so I hoped.

Madeleine did care for her mother but found the experience so wearing that, on my return, to my dismay she seemed almost distraught. The following letter is what she wrote to our GP.

Sunday July 3rd, 2011

Dear Dr May,

My apologies for another interruption in your busy day. I returned home to Tasmania on Friday of last week after spending time with Mum and it is quite evident she is getting worse not better. There has been no obvious change with the Risperdal although I acknowledge it is still early days. Dad is so overwhelmed by it all he does not know which way to turn. She has threatened suicide by taking tablets.

As we discussed on Monday, Mum is constantly troubled by the false thoughts that Dad has been having an affair with someone. The story varies. Sometimes I was there, sometimes my brother was there, but neither of us knows what she is talking about. If I was not in the room with them Mum would immediately launch into a continuous barrage of questions and accusations whenever Dad comes in. Last night he could not cope alone and rang my brother at 0300 to come up to Skye to see if he could settle her. My brother spent three hours with her until dawn. I rang the following morning and was asked the same question I have been asked during every phone call I have had from her over the last three months or so: 'Was I there when she went into this woman's house and saw Dad?' She rang my brother four times, my sister-in-law four times, with the same question yesterday, seemingly unable to recall the answers or even the conversation. I am ashamed to say that I dread to hear the phone ring. Our family is in crisis. She wakes him at night to ask him these questions. He is reluctant to go out for fear that she will accuse him of being out with 'her'. The cruel thing is that she accuses him of this even when he has been sitting by her side for the whole of the evening. He has started to withdraw socially. She is no longer looking after herself or the house. She goes out in dirty clothes without caring. She will constantly come back to the accusations when even the most unrelated conversation starts up. We try to distract her as much as possible with other things but it is enormously draining. It is a reflection of Dad's enormous love for her when he says that he can cope with the constant abuse for as long as it takes for her to get better. I am not sure he understands or wants to understand the nature of multi-infarct dementia. He has denied she has a significant problem for eighteen months or so, covering for her socially. He is now entirely responsible for getting her medication on a daily basis.

She has now threatened to sell the family home and move out. This varies as well. Sometimes it is Dad who is moving out 'to live with his girlfriend' sometimes she wants to buy a smaller house and live there. I don't know any more. Mum continues to order goods from the TV shopping channel. We have carton loads of Tupperware, numerous shredders, blenders, grillers, makeup and jewellery jammed into drawers around the house. Needless to say they are haemorrhaging cash. Dad quietly takes them all down to the Salvation Army each week.

Having said all this there are fleeting periods (usually after hours of reassurance) when she is more lucid and settled. She is adamant that she can still handle all the financial dealings of the household. I have paid a couple of large VISA card bills for them over the last twelve months that had been overlooked. She tends to open mail and then just pile the bills/rubbish/letters on the kitchen bar. Dad has taken to going through them with her. This is the first time he has had to get involved with this in fifty years of marriage. Mum has always had a fear 'of going barmy' and regards mental illness and the need for psychiatric care as a weakness of character.

I have asked Dad to make an appointment to come and see you. He has no experience with dementia or mental illness issues. As you are aware he is an intensely private and stoic gentleman. The fact that he is no longer coping is deeply troubling to me. He will defend her to the hilt and could never conceive of doing anything to hurt her.

I wonder if it is time for an urgent ACAT referral as Dad is going to need more help as soon as possible. I know I am far too close to this situation to make any decent clinical decisions so I can only thank you again for your help.

Best wishes,

Dr Madeleine Wilcock (née Roe)

Madeleine's visit and her letter jump-started events. Instead of being a relatively private affair Ella's predicament now moved under the auspices of the public health system. That it was to a large degree taken out of my amateurish hands was no doubt an inevitable and proper development. That did not make the process any less distressing for either of us.

First came the Critical Assessment Team who judged, correctly, that we required more assistance, Ella in particular. A domestic carer came in for several mornings a week to provide help and a supervisor was appointed to observe my wife's health and symptoms. Then came two interviews with consultant physicians in geriatric health. This was in mid-2011 and in one of the consulting rooms I was to hear for the first time the words 'Alzheimer's Disease'. The letter is still with me. It says ominously: 'Principal diagnosis: Benign Memory Impairment versus Early Alzheimer's Disease.' The physician showed me microscope images revealing traces of brain cells being destroyed.

Presumably as a consequence of the observations there came a truly dreadful day, dreadful for Ella and without much doubt the worst day of my entire life, to that date, possibly with a chance of retaining its standing. We were told that Ella needed to have her mental impairment further investigated, the first step being an assessment in the Royal Adelaide Hospital. It was made clear that this was compulsory, which, although the necessity was clear enough, had implications I didn't much want to contemplate. What else would soon be compulsory?

Though I had tried to explain the appointment she had forgotten about it when the team arrived, consisting, if I remember correctly, of the team leader, the supervisor, a psychiatrist and two nurses. In addition there were two policemen who were considerate enough to keep a very low profile and did not enter the house at all. When asked why they were there they told me that some patients resisted so strenuously that their authority and physical assistance were required. In fact both seemed decent individuals who would have much preferred doing something other than restraining elderly ladies.

As it was, when Ella realised, probably in a fragmented sort of way, that she was going to be taken into a psychiatric hospital she refused utterly to go. When the team leader persisted (what else could he do?) she fled down the long corridor of our house, sobbing and screaming hysterically, attempting to escape into the garden at the back.

She had dressed very smartly, perhaps believing this was to be some social occasion. And what did I do? Exactly nothing. Whether there was anything that actually could be done was problematic but the policemen must have guessed my self-contempt and internal rage because one said quietly: 'Sir, don't.'

I've tried to shake this memory out of my mind where it lies like some revolting stain. Not that there was anything useful to be done, other than a strong determination to appoint myself to be close beside her for the rest of her or my life. Every day of it. I'm very sorry if this sounds a sanctimonious sort of statement. It isn't meant to be.

Beckett's characters in *Waiting for Godot* put it in perspective.

> *Vladimir:* We are not saints but we have kept our appointment. How many people can boast as much?
> *Estragon:* Billions.

And there'll be billions more, parents, husbands, wives, brothers, sisters, children, friends, keeping their appointments at the care homes where the Alzheimers' sufferers fade away.

At this point the demon nightmare was coming often, rarely allowing seven nights to pass without its pointless unequal struggle. Yet how much worse could it have been had the creature attacked Ella, or so I thought, before eventually grasping that in reality it had done so. When my wife sometimes appeared in the dream, she always stayed in our palatial dream-house. If only reality could have replicated the illusion.

The crisis team gathered clothes and nightwear and we departed in a convoy to the hospital. She was placed in a smallish room with three beds. One was vacant, in the other was a young man, also mentally impaired. His father was sitting alongside him. The father and I recognised each other at once. He had been a member of 5B, my very first class at St Peter's College, thirty-eight years earlier. My heart went out to father and son. Why wasn't my one-time pupil out watching his son play Aussie Rules? Or going fishing together? Or playing tennis in the park. And lighting up the barbecue afterwards? It wasn't that much to ask for, was it?

There were three days of tests for Ella, even briefly one for me. It was explained to me that she was suffering from dementia, though apparently unclear as yet whether it was multi-infarct dementia or Lewy's Body dementia, or Alzheimer's Disease, or vascular dementia, or Binswanger's Disease. The words were meaningless, like 'Dachau' chalked on a railway wagon.

The eventual recommendation was for further tests to be undertaken at Rosewood, a department of Glenside Psychiatric Hospital. It had earlier been known as Parkside Lunatic Asylum, which is more or less how I'd thought of it. We seemed to be sinking deep, but if so we'd go down together. She must not face this alone.

Rosewood was a small, single-storey, pre-fabricated sort of place, overshadowed by the looming Victorian monolith of the original Glenside Hospital. Ella was a patient there in late 2011 for about seven weeks. The days repeated one another closely. Usually about eleven o'clock there was an interview with one of the specialists. Thereafter the day was more or less free. One of the psychiatrists, a young Indian, was prepared to listen to my questions. To my despair he told me that the obsession with infidelity was incurable. He added that in his experience more than half of his married patients had that particular delusion. Another common misconception was that of one partner secretly pilfering the family's savings. So if the obsession with infidelity was incurable, then the tactic of hanging on gamely, accepting the bad times and waiting for our luck to turn, was a self-deceiving fallacy. So where did that leave us?

Well, it left us exactly where Santiago, the old fisherman, found himself in Hemingway's *The Old Man and the Sea.*

He was an old man who fished alone in a skiff in the Gulf Stream and he had gone eighty-four days now without taking a fish. But after about forty days without a fish the boy's parents had told him that the old man was now definitely and finally salao, which is the worst form of unlucky...

Like us the old man's luck had run out. So what could he do? Same as us. Keep trying. What else is left to do?

I was determined that no day should see her alone and as few as possible away from her home. So the days built up a pattern. They would start about ten o'clock when we would walk together round the drab grounds of the hospital, waiting for that morning's appointment, usually stopping briefly at a down-at-heel café where silent customers stared at us, the tradesmen with indifference, keeping their distance, as one might from lepers, the inmates with a lopsided peering, and occasional questions, or rather one question occasionally: 'What's the matter with you?' This seemed generally addressed to me and it was tempting to ask, 'How long have you got?' The morning interview over, we would go out for lunch. Usually this was an opportunity, particularly when we were driving, for the fusillade of accusations to be repeated. Always it was the same threadbare, hackneyed dialogue. Anger, sarcasm, and particularly humour were all out of the question as responses, leaving only the draining cross-examination:

'Have you seen her today?'

'No, I haven't.'

'Did you see her yesterday?'

'No, I didn't.'

Eventually the close presence of other people would end the futile catechisms and in company, in a restaurant for instance, we would talk together, often quite normally. The same applied in the ward's lounge or common room where about a dozen people, mostly middle-aged or elderly ladies, looked passively at a television screen which seemed to display very little other than unlikely advertisements, one for hotel rooms in Los Angeles appearing to be a particular favourite.

There were several incidents from the time at Rosewood. I would prefer to have forgotten all of them. Firstly was her phone call to Gina. She had found the correct number in the ward's directory. What was said remains unknown to me. It must have come as a grotesque surprise to the lady concerned. The implications didn't bear thinking about. Perhaps Gina thought that I'd boasted about such an affair, a scenario that made me cringe. My feeble reaction, I'm ashamed to say, was to do nothing. About six months later Ella repeated the call. This time I asked my son to contact the lady and apologise, and was deeply grateful when he did.

The ward's administration seemed uncertain how long visitors could stay. My intention was to stay as long as possible, which generally meant about eight o'clock in the evening. I would then say goodbye to Ella and go to the car. To my horror Ella would somehow emerge from the ward and bar my way, screaming that she was coming with me. She would fling herself on the car's bonnet, until I got out and accompanied her back into the ward. This sequence would replay itself three or four times an evening. There never seemed to be any helpers around. Eventually I persuaded her to go to bed and sat until she went to sleep. The other lady with whom she shared a room would on occasion announce that my presence was unwanted and would be reported to the authorities. In the long-gone happy days my response would have been: 'Good lady, I answer only to a higher authority.' But the time for laughter was over, almost certainly forever. This sad business with the car happened on a number of evenings. The sense of betrayal as I drove away never left me.

Nor did it end there. Once on leaving her my distress was so overwhelming that while driving home in the twilight my mind ceased to function properly, nor did it return to reality before there was a crackling, snapping sort of noise, exactly the noise I'd heard twice previously when crashing through the scrub and undergrowth to avoid the terrorists' ambushes on Rhodesian backroads. Fortunately there was no serious collision on this suburban Adelaide road other than with two staked saplings which then lay there uprooted. I sat in the car for half an hour or so, reluctant to drive on lest the same coma effect returned. A few days later came a fine for having driven through a red light on that same

According to the psychiatrists of Rosewood Ella would not get better. According to me she would. I loved her, therefore she would. It would take time but, as with Hemingway's old fisherman, unless one gives up there is no defeat.

In fact I believed the psychiatrists' positions and my own both to be true, thus qualifying for Scott Fitzgerald's accolade: 'The test of a first-rate intelligence is the ability to hold two opposed ideas in mind at the same time and still retain the ability to function.' Certainly there were two opposed ideas held in my mind; it was the ability to function about which there was a good deal of doubt. Driving blindly into trees, vomiting in gardening stores, weeping in a paralysis on a golf course – none of these suggested a highly functioning mind. Thus the equation had to rule out the 'first-rate intelligence'. Chastening as realism usually is it didn't bother me a lot, there being other things to think about.

Memories from this time, the time of the carers, provided they don't hurt, are available but usually not relevant to this story. Whenever possible we went to watch our grandchildren play cricket. We took deck chairs and found shade under the gum trees of scorched suburban grounds or the plane trees lining St Peter's College's lawns. Out in the middle Rob and Alex batted on, sometimes to centuries, but always to their gran's approval. Quite often she would remark: 'Alex stands just like you stood' and for those brief moments we seemed back at long-ago places. 'Do you remember Eastbourne?' she would say. Remember it? Walking on the esplanade with her, the sea smooth lace-fringed emerald, her laughter at saucy postcards on the pier, young and in love in the sea-scented air. Or Elsham. Do you remember Elsham? Holding hands in the dusk, the grass webbed with dew, swallows swirling along the white boundary line, brushing just above the grass; in the twilight bats zig-zagging sketchily above our heads, as the players leave.

'Goodbye, Mick. Goodbye, Jim. Thanks for the game.'

'And thank Mrs Stanley for the tea,' said Ella, nudging my arm.

As 2013 came and went, my wife's physical health deteriorated. She was taking what seemed a vast amount of medication. Perhaps it was effective as she seemed calmer and the tedious accusations of the previous two or so years became less frequent and somehow less manic. The mysterious 'fat woman', for instance, disappeared from the narrative. The nights with the 'sundowner effect' were still bad, but during the day hours could pass without more than the occasional absent-minded barb. Also she was putting on considerable weight, now weighing substantially more than I did since the stresses had stripped away so much of my physique.

Now she had a number of falls, or to be accurate not quite falls but more a case of her muscles failing to deal with her weight, so that she slid off chairs or slumped to the floor when getting out of bed. On each occasion I had to raise her up and since she lacked the strength to help it was a demanding task. Nevertheless on every occasion but one (of which more later) and there were many, my prayer (always the same) was answered. It went something like this: 'Let me be young and strong again. Just for a few seconds. Just this once.' It seemed to work, though defying logic.

For some reason Ella never really liked showering and throughout our marriage far preferred to have a hot bath. She persisted in the bad years but as she grew weaker the task of lifting her upright in the bath and lifting her out was not easy, though something I was happy to do.

What was the driving force in the latter years of her illness (particularly 2014 and 2015) was my certainty that this was the time of trial, that everything in my life had in a strange way prepared me for this. Life, that had always been relatively easy, now would be different. It would be hard and it would hurt, for both of us, but here was the moment. It had come. The fun and pleasure and joy were over. But she needed me and that was more than enough.

I felt as if I were walking with destiny and that all my life had been but a preparation for this hour and this trial.

The voice is Winston Churchill's and the hour is 1940, but the words struck a chord, nor did I feel, where our future was concerned, that they were in any way inappropriate.

XXVI

2013 brought a newish experience for me, a visit to a psychiatrist. This ran against all my preconceptions, as to my regret I was not asked to do a Rorschach test and interpret ink-blots. Our entire discussion was based on my loss of weight and the likelihood that this would have serious effects on my health. It was disturbingly reminiscent of Heinrich Hoffman's cautionary tale of Augustus, a chubby lad who so adamantly refused his mother's soup that in four days 'he scarcely weighed a sugar plum', and soon:

He's like a little bit of thread
And on the fifth day he was dead'

The psychiatrist's argument that disturbed me more than this hypothetical ultra-wasting away was that my medical care for Ella would be compromised, thus would it not be better for both of us were she to be found a place in a Care Home? It was explained that in such a Home she would receive professional medical care, along with proper monitoring of temperature, blood pressure and so on. Our own GP would visit and supervise her treatment. Eventually and reluctantly I consented and went home to face what experience told me would be a barrage of abuse and accusations on the grounds that, as soon as she was incarcerated in care, Gina would move into our house. Had it not been for the insistence of the Assessment Team's supervisor I'd have gladly scrapped the whole notion.

Places in reputable Homes were not easy to find, I was informed, but one came up in an outlying suburb. It was known, rather grandly, as The Viceroy and situated in Golden Grove (an area presumably called after one of the ships of the First Fleet, that had reached Australia in 1788). Like schools and hotels, care residences are bound to differ from one another. The Viceroy struck me as a commercial, no-frills set-up, doing enough to satisfy primary requirements, though the residents seemed to be there for the sake of the organisation rather than the reverse.

Whenever I visited (i.e. virtually every day) the staff all appeared to have changed from the previous day, nor did most appear to have a name, though several displayed badges of various sorts, e.g. 'Administrator' or 'Counsellor'. Ella's room was functional enough, though she never knew where it was, a memory failure that always occurred whatever the place in which she was a resident. Our supervisor, who was still responsible for her, did not seem impressed by our Golden Grove experience, and after three weeks there she was transferred to the Helping Hand Care Home in North Adelaide.

For a brief period around Christmas she did come home and I suppose it was a last desperate attempt to put off the inevitable separation, which shows how much I had yet to learn of Alzheimer's. Our supervisor had to tell me bluntly that my scrambling efforts would eventually make things worse. By now I knew how a rat in a trap felt, though that's only putting it mildly, since the rat, though doubtless feeling steadily worse, may well by its nature never experience that total despair that seems humanity's unique penalty. Somehow rats think they'll make it, in the fashion of Santiago, the old man of Hemingway's tale, though Hemingway himself was less convincing when, contrary to his own rhetoric, he opted to blow his brains out. The rat wouldn't do that and nor would I, particularly not while my wife was relying on me. Anyway what would our grandchildren have thought of me?

Still vestiges of the double belief clung on: things will get better and things will not get better. But it was worse than that: having faith that things will get better while fearing they won't is perfectly normal. My version was brutally polarised and, as it turned out, false, there being a third option, as you will see.

I recall clearly another and very different feeling. This would happen for a few seconds while waking in the morning, still drowsy and not yet even half-aware, before an unwelcome consciousness told me exactly what the regimented day would be, that is the same as every other day. But just for a few moments before my subconscious engaged with reality it would deal me a flash-back so poignant that, like Caliban, I wished not to have woken, but to be dreaming still.

This recurring reverie placed me with my brothers and a couple of small friends paddling in a stream (we always called it 'the beck') that ran through poppied fields of barley, owned by my father on one side and my uncle on the other. It was green-lit under arching ash trees, and we would delight in the clear rippling water, half way to our knees, the pebbles mossed and smooth underfoot, minnows and sticklebacks darting around our toes. 'Remember to take water-cress home for Mum,' said someone, either my younger brother or Pan in Arcadia.

After a week at home Ella moved into residence at the Helping Hand Aged Care home in Buxton Street, North Adelaide. It had accommodation for 155 people. The large majority were elderly people, who were not ill but finding it difficult to live lives without organised help, and there were smaller sections such as palliative care or dementia care. I got to know it very well as Ella was to be there from January 2014 until her death in December 2015.

Helping Hand had much to recommend it in various ways. The accommodation was comfortable and the meals provided certainly acceptable, though necessarily institutional. Almost all (but not quite all) the staff were, as one would expect, competent, with several admirable ladies for whom I had nothing but praise. There was a well-designed garden where Ella and I often sat together, a cheerful café, a library, a chapel where we regularly attended services, a gift shop, a craft shop, and a hair salon, which Ella liked, where her hair was done weekly.

Another favourable factor was the location. The building is in Buxton Street close to Wellington Square and the surrounding streets are pleasant to walk in, with numerous late-Victorian sandstone or bluestone dwellings often with attractive gardens. O'Connell Street, which is lively and has plenty of restaurants and shops, is quite close. The whole area became utterly familiar to us.

So much for the bricks and mortar. T.S. Eliot's poem *Journey of the Magi* describes the difficult journey the kings had to Bethlehem, with cold weather in the dead of winter, refractory camels, the villages dirty and charging high prices, so much so that the kings regretted leaving their summer palaces and the silken girls bringing sherbet. But they reached the stable and their venture 'was (you may say) satisfactory'. It's an interesting ninety per cent sort of approval, and to a considerable extent our opinions of both Helping Hand and North Adelaide were pretty much the same.

However, the environs were not the heart of the matter by any means. In the case of Helping Hand there were the clients and staff, these dividing into denominations: there were those in palliative care that one never met, there were two wards of dementia patients, these comprising about twenty-five people, and also there were those, much more numerous, who resided there for care and company. The clientele seemed disproportionately female and frequently members of this third group were to be found playing bridge or mahjong, or simply chatting with visitors in the café-cum-dining room. Ella liked me to sit with her among these cheerful get-togethers and often we would have morning tea there. For the residents (for want of a better word) there was a variety of activities. For instance, Tuesday was film afternoon, Wednesday was classical music, and on Thursdays there was entertainment, usually a sort of concert. One afternoon we had the Adelaide Male Voice Choir and I was pleased to meet my golf partner among the singers.

The dementia patients could, if they wished, come to any of these occasions and in audiences of around fifty or sixty were virtually indistinguishable, particularly as so many of both groups were in wheelchairs. A memorable afternoon, still vivid in my mind, developed at one of these events. The entertainer was a pianist, and a remarkably talented one, who visited several times. She played in a vivacious, non-stop, music-hall style, this no doubt being, very properly, for our benefit, as our average age was probably around eighty and we all knew the words of Vera Lynn's 'Wish me luck as you wave me goodbye'. The pianist asked us to name tunes we would like to hear and sing to, so we had 'Daisy Bell' and 'Goodbye, Dolly Gray' and I held Ella's hand, among old ladies eighteen again and irresistible, at least in the imagination of their hearts.

One moment, though, was deeply sad. A lady from Ella's ward requested 'Tipperary' and our pianist duly obliged, then strummed a few chords awaiting a further request. The same lady requested: 'Could you play "It's a long way to Tipperary"?' The pianist paused, smiled, said (I can hear her saying it), 'It's a nice tune, Mary', and played it again. A pause. I swear I knew what was coming. It did. Different lady but same request: 'Could you play "Tipperary"?' Ella and I were adjacent to the piano. The pianist, glassy-eyed, looked in my direction. Or for my direction. 'Play it,' I said. 'What else is there to do?'

We never missed Thursdays. They were generally entertaining and off-beat; once it was a so-called Mexican trio in enormous hats, shaking maracas and singing 'Manana, manana, is soon enough for me' and 'South of the border, down Mexico way' pronouncing Mexico as Me-he-co, which convinced no-one, particularly as their professional title was The Christies Beach Ensemble.

Don't let me underplay it: the show was fine, almost as memorable as another unforgettable afternoon, this time a different pianist who sang as she played, running through a 1940-ish repertoire. There must have been a sprinkling of ninety-year-olds in the audience who remembered the war years as their years, as there was a semi-spontaneous outbreak of period pieces such as 'Kiss me good night Sergeant-major' and, with a gesture towards the universality of war, Marlene Dietrich's 'Underneath the lamplight by the barracks gate'.

However the supreme moment was about to come, as a tiny ancient man rose and sang unaccompanied that superbly meaningless lyric:

A soldier was saying goodbye to
his horse,
Saying goodbye to his horse,

> *And as he was saying goodbye to his horse,*
> *He was saying goodbye to his horse.*

The thought struck me that Samuel Beckett would never have bothered to write *Waiting for Godot* had he ever previously come across this mantra. I had heard it once before when a friend told me it was the battle-song of Charlton Athletic FC, which seemed almost too good to be true. The ancient man croaked out, 'Come on, all together,' but a nurse said, 'Thank you, Clarence.' Gallantly he began the second verse, which is actually identical with the first, as is the third.

'Thank you very much, Mr Crabtree,' the matron herself intervened. I was sorry. I would have liked to sing the song.

Unexpectedly my chance would come a few weeks later. A different pianist, same sort of occasion. She was playing songs from *Oh, what a lovely war.* Some were familiar and people joined in, but then she played the first bars of 'Chanson de Craonne'. There was silence. This French song was so profoundly antiestablishment that it was banned in France from 1917 until 1974 and a reward of a million francs was offered, without success, to anyone revealing its composer. (Hopeless, of course! After all who composed 'Saying goodbye to his horse'?)

'Do you know it?' the pianist asked me. As usual Ella had positioned her wheelchair next to the piano. 'Nobody else seems to.'

'I do,' I said. 'Well, only the chorus.'

'Sing it,' she said.

'I'm a pretty hopeless singer.'

'Can you speak French?'

'Yes.'

'Then we'll sing it together.'

'Just the chorus then.'

Adieu la vie, adieu l'amour,
Adieu toutes les femmes,
C'est bien fini, c'est pour toujours
...

You've got the idea, I'm sure. Life, love, girls, it's all over, for always.

Car nous sommes tous condamnés
Nous sommes les sacrifiés.

The listeners in the ever-present wheel-chairs, grey heads drooping, eyes fading, behind tortoise-shell glasses, lost husbands and wives already over the unreachable horizon, seemed not unapproving, though probably already thinking of afternoon tea. '*Vous êtes les sacrifiés.*'

Here and there moments came when one almost smiled, but one never laughed. Laughter in the dementia wards was unknown. Its absence saddened me, as did my sorrow for these people whom the demon was blowing away like chaff in numbers that would before long, if they had not already done so, dwarf the death toll of Craonne, or Chemin des Dames as it is now often called. Chemin des Dames? Road of the ladies! And one of the ladies was my wife.

She must be spared at all costs both the loneliness and the sense of confinement that so many of her fellow patients must have felt before they slipped into a sort of detached inertia. Once swallowed by this abyss there would be no returning.

My objectives were firstly, to be with her every day as far as possible and, secondly, to try to make each day different and at least part of the day spent outside the ward's walls. Whether this was medically sound, I'm unsure. In the years 2014 and 2015, with the exception of two brief visits to my daughter in Tasmania and a rushed business trip to England, every day was spent with her. The times varied from twenty-four hours to three hours, the latter being only on Saturdays when generally I watched or coached the soccer games of Saints Old Scholars. Every other activity went out of the window. Cricketing Saturdays were different as we always went together to watch our grandchildren play. 'The soul is healed by being with children,' wrote Dostoevsky, rightly. I was reading a lot of Dostoevsky about this time, though all that Russian melancholy was exactly what I didn't need. In October 2017 the Federal Aged Care Minister, Ken Wyatt, in a speech to the National Press Club made this comment: 'I have heard that up to forty per cent of people in residential aged care have no visitors

365 days of the year.' That's right. No visitors. None at all. It sounds unbelievable.

Lest you make the error of proposing my actions as those of a would-be saint let me say that, overwhelmingly, there was no other action and destination I would have preferred other than to be walking into the ward, longing to see her and to tell her our plans for the day.

Always, until the events of June 2015 (more later!) made it impossible, she would ask to be taken home. The medical team were happy for this to happen for spells of two days each week so, usually on a Sunday morning, equipped with medication, we would leave to spend forty-eight hours together at home. She was by this time much less aggressively accusatory, her medication presumably calming her. Indeed there were nights when, in bed, she would push vigorously across complaining that it was cold on her side, and then her presence made the long happy shared years seem near enough to touch.

The days were divided between time spent in the wards and time outside. Let's deal with the outside first. Almost every day she was dressed and ready to leave Helping Hand by eleven o'clock at the latest. We would then drive out, simply looking at the city, before deciding on lunch at one of her favourite restaurants, among them Mount Osmond Golf Club, Sorelle's on Magill Road, the German Arms in Hahndorf, or the nearby Wellington Hotel. Sometimes we drove down to the coast where she liked the Stamford Grand and the cluster of cafes around Henley Square.

Gradually and sadly she was both weakening and putting on weight and, though short walks of thirty yards or so were feasible, it was necessary to pack a wheelchair into the car for most outings. She liked to be pushed through Botanic Park (another favourite restaurant) or through the grounds of St Peter's College, or along the esplanades and piers of Glenelg or Henley Beach, and sometimes along Rundle Mall where on the right days we could find entertaining buskers or jugglers. One morning there was the Australian Ladies Hockey team, radiating vigour and gloss. 'I was like that once,' she said.

There were some odd, not to say grotesque, incidents, two taking place in ladies' toilet rooms. The first occurred at the Regal Cinema where we had just watched *The Second-best Exotic Marigold Hotel* after which Ella went to the toilet. There was a delay so I went to the door and called out, 'Are you all right?'

'No. I'm stuck. I can't get up.'

The cubicle was such that she had no hand-hold to lift herself and from a seated position could not reach the lock. There was a crowd waiting in the foyer for the next show and the man dishing out tickets said he was too busy to help, but directed me to a cupboard where there was a small step-ladder. The only hope, he said, was to climb up, reach over the door and release the bolt. A number of ladies using the facility gazed, then looked away. What they thought I cannot imagine. Theirs not to reason why, perhaps. The space between the door top and the ceiling was narrow and my only hope was to slide head-first through this gap and somehow cope with the subsequent fall. I got lucky, collecting only bruises, and that was that. Regrettably no lady asked me what I thought I was doing since there were so many available answers, such as 'Practising for the Olympic gymnastics, horizontal bar event' or 'Searching for the lost treasure of Sierra Madre'.

The second incident though not altogether dissimilar, lacked any redeeming element whatever. This time it was a café toilet and another cry for help from Ella. This time she opened the door of the cubicle and to my horror I saw her legs and the floor were daubed with semi-liquid faeces. Carefully I cleaned her, glad that her clothes had not been soiled, took her back into the café and found her a seat and a cup of coffee before returning to the toilet. I then cleaned the floor and without being able to find anything helpful like a brush or a pan, used my hands and paper to scoop the faeces into the bowl. What struck me at the time was how little it meant. If my wife needed my help then it brought neither indignity nor embarrassment. It was nothing. Less than nothing.

One sad day in May 2015 she got out of the car and fell on the road. Her body was so limp I could neither lift her back into the car or onto the wheelchair. Fortunately Helping Hand was nearby and nurses brought out a sort of lifting mechanism that raised her enough to be installed in her wheelchair. Thankfully this happened on a quiet street and close to the Home. It meant our driving days were over and for the five months before her death our excursions all took place with my wheeling her. We went many miles through the streets of North Adelaide. Ella's favourite destination was O'Connell Street, which was always busy and cheerful. We knew every restaurant and coffee shop and, for that matter, every other place on the street. There was a supermarket and a book shop through which she particularly liked to perambulate, if that's the word.

She was heavy and the chair was, to be kind, basic. Eventually we knew every paving stone in the suburb. Some stones were smooth, neatly joined and level. Others were crooked or uneven. The kerbside inclines designed for handicapped people's chairs were sometimes helpful, but others had to be avoided at all costs. Ella liked reading the blue plaques that were on quite a number of houses in the area, e.g. 'these bluestone residences on land granted to James Solomon,' or 'area made accessible by horse-trams: 1878.'

St Laurence's Church was cool and still. We often went in and lit candles. She liked to pause under jacaranda trees to look up and marvel at their blueness, or pause under the flight path of aircraft so low they cast shadows on us. 'What keeps them up?' she would say, but I've never really had a convincing answer for that.

Towards the end she was unable to sit upright and instead of a chair had a sort of mattress on wheels. This was heavy and unwieldy but we still went out into the warmth of the spring sunshine and the cool of the breeze, if only to be alone and alive together.

XXVII

Inside the wards where Ella lived for two years was an organisation, one of many in similar places, that may never generate an appropriate literature. Bereft of any ability to think or write dispassionately one can only speculate which great writer would observe this society and with his or her own unique perception do justice to the sacrifiés. Dickens? Orwell? Maybe Solzhenitsyn or Dostoevsky who both knew what it was like to be interned, not that the hardships of Russian labour camps remotely resembled Helping Hand. Ken Kesey's novel *One Flew Over the Cuckoo's Nest* was on the right lines. Eventually though it came down to an unlikely cross between Dickens' humanity and Kafka's nihilism.

Inside the wards were three categories of people: staff, patients and visitors. In general the staff were good people, competent in a difficult profession, and coping well with what could be draining situations. I thank them, with one notable exception. Ella loved rings. Her favourite was her wedding ring. She fell while in the ward and her hand was so swollen that the ring had to be sawn off. I took it to a jeweller I knew who told me that the ring's gold was of such high quality that he could not find any in Adelaide for its repair. If we could wait for a while he would find appropriate metal from interstate or overseas. So he did, and the ring was restored to Ella. A week or so later it was no longer on her hand, nor was her opal ring. The opal had been my present for some bygone birthday. The ring it decorated had been designed and made in silver by Ella herself as part of her Fine Arts diploma.

'Where are your rings?' I asked.

'Someone took them off.'

'Who?'

'I don't know. A nurse.'

No-one seemed able to help, however high in the organisation, but a junior nurse spoke to me when we found ourselves alone: 'Try looking in the local pawn shops,' she said. I did. There were several not far away. Some proprietors co-operated, others did not, until I asked to use their phones to speak to the police. Schoolmasters have unexpected allies. Two of my most formidable pupils had become policemen, and clearly both had learned (presumably at the Police Academy) to favour the first person plural: 'Not trying to be unhelpful, are we, sir?' Even they had no success. I bought another wedding ring, in appearance at least not dissimilar to the first, and Ella seemed to forget the affair though once or twice wondering where her opal was.

Both of Ella's wards, where dementia cases were cared for, were of necessity kept permanently locked. The locks were numerically coded in a sequence of numbers that regularly I forgot, but my abiding memory of the doors is how inmates would wait for me to open them and then try to dash out, forcing me to bar the way, while hating every moment of it. One lady foxed me by wearing a smart suit and equally smart hat while carrying a suitcase. Her escape terminated in the garden and nurses escorted her back as she wept uncontrollably. 'Why won't you let me see my husband?' she sobbed. I felt weak and inadequate.

Ella's first ward, Frome, had a diverse group of inmates, while her second, Garden Court, was much quieter with about eight or nine mostly elderly ladies, almost all being quiet and withdrawn. Frome was different. How different was illustrated on day one when a patient slid past my feet and along the corridor on his stomach, seal-like, touching the skirting-boards with outstretched fingers. He was, it turned out, both demented and blind, a notable triumph for the demon.

The staff worked hard and I admired them for it, but in Frome Ward the psychic currents never let up. One gentleman, who never appeared from his room, could be heard bellowing again and again like a tormented bull. It was hard to reconcile that his son had been one of my pupils at Saints, and that we must have met socially or perhaps on parent evenings. When his wife visited we always spoke of the school.

A middle-aged man, whose father was in care, appeared never to leave the ward. The father seemed paralysed, always slumped in a chair. At meal-times the son would feed him meticulously, one careful spoonful after another, urging him to swallow: 'Must keep your strength up, Dad.'

Then there was another pair, possibly husband and wife, but more likely brother and sister as there was a strong facial resemblance. The lady was always with him, coaxing him to eat, taking him for walks in the nearby streets, an avatar of devotion. I missed very few days in almost two years; she missed none, as far as I could tell.

There was one moment of numbing dismay. It was morning as I entered the ward to see my friend, Donald Guthrie, standing there. He was as ever immaculate in a blue pin-striped suit. Upright and handsome, he stood straight-backed like the top-class South African rugby player he had once been, though his red hair had now faded to grey. His son had been at Saints and later a player in teams I had coached and Dr Guthrie had for a time been our soccer club medic.

Whom was he visiting? I walked across and shook his hand. He looked at me perplexed and I recognised the chilling incomprehension that every ward patient, except at times Ella herself, had in common. One happy evening we had been to dinner at his house, swapping our stories of Rhodesia for his of South Africa. Now all that was left, as we stood in the ward's foyer, were my fumbling attempts to connect: 'John Roe, you remember? I taught your boy, Angus.' He looked away, my words left hanging in the air like a fly droning.

Ella made no friends in either of her two wards, but among the dementia sufferers, as far as I could tell, neither did anyone else. In the wards was a collection of inward-looking strangers, none of whom seemed capable of connecting or sympathising with any other. Frequently, when I arrived, her opening words were an imperative: 'Take me out of here.' Even when she was permanently restricted to a wheelchair, in the last six months of 2015, there would come the stern command to leave. When it was a cold, windy day outside or raining she would consent to being wheeled around the home's interior, often stopping at the café for tea, or in the library or gift shop, or even in the front porch to watch the rain.

The Via Dolorosa, the Way of Suffering, is about 600 metres long. It is a road that runs through Jerusalem, starting where Christ was sentenced, scourged and crowned with thorns, and ending at the hill of crucifixion, which at that time was outside the city walls but now has been over-built by the Church of the Holy Sepulchre. The dreadful walk had its own cruel reality, but has also acquired an aureole of images that may or may not be true, several having the look of the devotional literature of medieval Europe. Actual events and later images together mingle under the name of the Stations of the Cross. The number of Stations itself is variable but traditionally the first is Pilate's judgement and the last is Christ's death. The fourth Station was where Christ passed by his mother, the fifth marks Simon of Cyrene carrying the cross for a while, and the sixth was where Saint Veronica wiped the sweat and blood away from Christ's face, supposedly creating on the cloth a likeness of his features.

That Ella and every other sufferer of Alzheimer's disease travelled or are travelling the Via Dolorosa is indisputable. By the second decade of the 21st century it was very clear our luck had been exhausted. Any turn of events looked sure to be for the worse and before long they were. Stations three, seven and nine on the road to Golgotha were all similar. Each marked where Christ fell. On the road outside Helping Hand Ella fell. She had fallen inside the home, too, when her wedding ring had to be sawn off. Station nine, her third fall, was at Skye one night in June 2015. She fell awkwardly, trapped between a wardrobe and a bed, so that it was impossible for me to lift her to her feet, though I tried for an hour or more. Despairing I phoned for an ambulance. Even they had difficulties but eventually she was transported to the Royal Adelaide Hospital. When Christ went down for the third time he must have wondered whether he would ever get up again. Or, indeed, whether it was worth getting up with Golgotha ahead. We reached the hospital about 1.00am. The day had twenty-three hours to go. It was one of the two worst days of my life. Perhaps my future still holds one worse but I seriously doubt that. 'If two people love one another there can be no happy end to it.' Dostoevsky again.

I don't want to write about that day. I just don't want to! But since it's got to be done it can wait its turn and we'll just sit on the roadside together for a while, my beautiful girl and I, and reminisce, and the crowd and the centurions can do as they please.

XXVIII

Our home of forty years was high on the slopes of the Mount Lofty range that overlooks the city of Adelaide. The position and the views it allows are liberating in their vastness and variety. As Ella reminded me occasionally, with a totally unjustified hint of domestic drudgery, she designed the house to ensure the finest view was from the kitchen windows. This was correct in a *primus inter pares* sort of way, as from other rooms and the garden's terraces a 180° panorama of sky, treetops, city and sea awaited us every day, bringing a sense of airy spaciousness that has never waned.

Below us Adelaide's far-reaching suburbs extend to the sea and the horizon, a confetti of white or pale-red rooftops sprinkling the darkish green expanse of trees. The multi-rise city centre lifts above the trees, inverted oblongs clustered and compressed, a child's building block creation. The immense blue dome of the air arches from the hills behind us to the distant sea ahead.

The sky itself is an endless delight, perfect both in summer's cobalt blue and in the eye-catching presence and passage of clouds. With Adelaide's prevailing westerlies the clouds come rolling up from the horizon on an air-built thoroughfare, arriving as if for our delighted inspection, before disappearing over the ranges behind us.

When the low misty rain-clouds come the city disappears and one sees only hazy veiled treetops and the merest suggestions of nearby roofs. Sometimes low clouds rub against our windows, and at other times one can look down upon altogether different formations, the main mass obscuring the city, but high above narrow grey bands with golden edges. The scope can be so wide on rainy days that there are separate columns of downward slanting grey lines, just as a child draws rain, so neatly outlined that one can distinguish which distant suburb has rain falling. There are times too when columns of light pour down from gaps in the cloud cover. The surprise delights: today, as I look out, there are rolling swathes of white, edged with an unpredictable rose-pink.

Following the eruption in 1815 of the Tambara volcano in Indonesia the world's sunsets changed, to be portrayed in the works of the great English artist, J.M.W. Turner and his contemporaries. After Krakatoa exploded in 1883 similar extravagant sunsets appeared. Paintings from both periods display the sky as a turbulent red-ochre. There are sunsets over Adelaide that deserve Turner and replicate, though possibly understated, Krakatoa's flamboyance. From our west-facing windows and terraces the evening skies are a generous display. When it's my turn to go and look at the dark I'll miss the many-coloured world, though I've seen it, and better still I saw it with Ella.

The night, of course, offered its own display. Beneath us lay a glitter of lights, white, amber, some vivid reds, laid out like a magic cloak. At times the lights sparkle and vibrate. Ella called them Joseph's Technicolour Dreamcoat, '...cream and crimson and silver and rose,' (plus fifty-three other colours according to Andrew Lloyd Webber).

There doesn't seem to be time to tell of the moon and the stars, since our sitting together on the side of the Via Dolorosa like this, talking about the sky, is a bit unrealistic. We'd better go on. Let me help you with the cross.

The dreadful journey had many hours left. The ambulance crew parked Ella's trolley along with another half-dozen patients, similarly waiting for day-break to come. It was a cold night. I recall fetching her extra blankets. Eventually the sound of traffic increased and morning brought rain streaking the windows. She was wheeled away and time passed, our daughter arriving in mid-morning having just flown in from Sydney.

Eventually the young doctor in charge appeared along with two of his equally youthful colleagues, they having conducted an intensive examination. I saw without surprise that he was an ex-pupil of mine, Dylan, this giving me a feeling that there was hope. Coincidences and luck have something in common. Or they did once.

We briefly recalled schooldays and his assistants looked at one another as we shook hands. 'In Adelaide,' said one, 'does everyone know everyone else?' Then came a hammer blow.

'She has Alzheimer's,' said Dylan, 'which you know, which is bad enough, but sadly I must tell you she has cancer as well.'

Our conversation was spasmodic, the diagnosis sending me into a state of semi-denial, a futile can-you-be-sure response.

'Where is the cancer?'

'In the bowel,' said Dylan.

'Can you remove it? Can you operate?'

'Yes, but...' He hesitated.

'What?'

The interview went on and on. In retrospect I sympathise with the young trio. How many times in their careers would they deliver similar grim verdicts? They looked boyish, still able to be upset.

My heart grew cold as he described the operation and colder still to hear of the consequences. In brief the surgery required would leave Ella with bowel incapacities that would make her life an indignity at best, a humiliation at worst, along with unavoidable pain, this all compounded by the misery of incomprehension that is Alzheimer's contribution.

'If you don't operate how long will my wife live?'

'Probably not more than a year. Perhaps six months.'

'And if you operate?'

'Probably longer. But with less quality of life.' Quality of life? As a phrase it sounded so everyday, run-of-the-mill, unexceptional, rather like 'palliative care'.

'Alzheimer's patients don't have much quality of life,' I said.

'I know,' said Dylan patiently.

'What do you advise?'

'I can't. Only you can decide.'

So I went and sat by myself in their private room and for a long time thought of our lives together and eventually did what I should have done earlier and asked what she would have done had it been I who was lost in an ignominious world of unremitting bewildered pain. Then I knew what to do.

The surgeons were waiting for me. In their sports jackets they reminded me of myself as a young schoolmaster. 'Do not operate,' I said.

They gathered around me, even shaking my hand. 'We were hoping you'd decide that way,' said one.

Maybe. Maybe they were just being kind. My daughter, too, told me I'd chosen rightly. It didn't feel that way. Maybe she was being kind. It felt more that my mind would always be congested with might-have-beens and indeed so it has been. It functions all right. I can prune roses and read the paper, but nothing has the slightest chance of obtaining my full attention. I'm always somewhere else: sitting alone in a leather armchair in a little room in the old Royal Adelaide Hospital, trying to do the right thing.

XXIX

So we returned to Helping Hand. Ella was moved from Frome Ward to Garden Court Ward, which she much preferred. The patients there were all quiet and reserved ladies, invariably polite. She made no friends but neither did anyone else, or so it appeared. But a change had come over her obsession with infidelity. This change had begun to emerge in the previous year, gradually at first, but as the months of 2014 passed by, so did the accusations seemingly exhaust themselves, until the taunts and allegations simply ceased. It was a paradox which baffles me still. At least the respite gave an opportunity to formulate my grief more adequately, the process removing some of its pain.

The nightmares of the demon became less frequent and less frenzied, even the action changing slightly: the glossy antiques establishment's two lower floors now seemed to have become part of our property and sometimes visitors were escorted around, admiring the exhibits, though they were never shown up to the third floor, it being still the domain of the demon. Curiously I seemed younger and less intimidated, even once or twice having the effrontery, *en passant,* to kick on its grey door.

Not that it was finished with me, or with my wife. When shortly after her death I was struggling through the complexities of probate our lawyer remarked that it was unusual to see only one partner in a marriage the sole owner of the family home.

'We owned it jointly,' I said.

'No. You relinquished your share of the ownership in 2012. Here's your signature.'

'I never signed that.'

'Then your name has been forged.'

The signature was not unlike mine, but I knew it for what it was: the demon's imprint. Its reptilian grasp would have been holding Ella's wrist.

'You monstrosity,' I thought. 'But they're coming for you. Not us, more likely our grandchildren or their children, but they've got your name, they know where you live. Like we dished it out to smallpox and rinderpest and polio. Remember them?'

Through the years of 2014 and 2015 my life simplified itself. Of the seven hundred and six days of those years before her death, there were in total sixteen days when I had no real choice but to be elsewhere. Of those years the remaining six hundred and ninety days and a good many nights we spent together. Her new calmness was welcome. As for the reasons one can only speculate. Perhaps she was slipping into the ultimate forgetfulness of Alzheimer's. With the erosion of memories those that had disappeared first were of the recent past, and they must have included the delusions that had tormented her so. It was as if she was reliving her life backwards, the further away in time the clearer and more comforting the memory. She liked to relate, happily and accurately, details from long ago, though occasionally there would come a touch of resentment invariably connected with recollections of her first marriage. Perhaps, too, my continued presence in itself reassured her, in that it clearly left me neither time nor inclination to be elsewhere with the imaginary Gina. This, though logical was probably unlikely. It made sense but in the Alzheimer's world making sense was a low priority.

A memory she recalled often and with affection was of our having dinner together in the theatre restaurant at Stratford-on-Avon, prior to watching *The Tempest.* 'We had lobster,' she would relate. 'Delicious, I'd never had it before. It was only when I first saw your overdraft that I realised who'd actually been paying for it.' Another vignette was the capture of the swarming bees at Grasby. The further back in time the clearer the recall: she related in detail the characters and idiosyncrasies of her teachers at South Park school. Another party trick was to describe the occupants of Walnut Place, running through the houses numerically, with an anecdote for each, for instance, at No.18 Peggy Nelson's baby had tragically drowned in the laundry tub. My favourite, and hers, I think, concerned a local boy, Ralph, who unpegged a tent which fell, enveloping Ella and other small girls who were occupying it. They emerged like the mythical Furies, and Ella herself set about the hapless Ralph as he fled to his parents' home, the girls then shrieking threats and invective from the gate.

Every day would be precious as the cancer was growing. Though she was physically fading she was, with the loss of weight, gradually coming to resemble her old self. In particular her facial features were now finer. Though her eyes, that had been cornflower blue, were now the paler blue of the horizon sky, they displayed again the challenging gaze of the enchantress who had bounced into the Tax Office's filing room, nineteen years old, mercurial and vivid in all her flashing femininity.

It was, as far as I remember, fairly late in 2014 that we were driving up to the Norton Summit hotel, where she liked to have afternoon tea. Something, a reminiscence perhaps, must have sparked the neuron circuits of her brain, for, from nowhere she said, 'I love you.' She smiled as she spoke, a queen returned from exile reinstated into her world, which, miraculously, had re-ordered itself. It had been four years at least, perhaps five, since I had heard those words, and had grown accustomed to thinking they would never be spoken again, they being the stuff dreams are made on.

> *To dream the impossible dream,*
> *To fight the unbeatable foe,*
> *To bear with unbearable sorrow,*
> *To run where the brave may not go...*

It's a great song, originally from the musical *Man of La Mancha,* in which Don Quixote, a knight errant chivalrously defending the helpless, usually finds his quests ending in comic failure. Today the song has shaken off any tincture of the comical, is indeed in tone almost heroic. My wife had had to bear with unbearable sorrow, all right, and had to fight an unbeatable foe.

And, of course, along with a great host of others, I'd learned to run where the brave may not go. Inside the dementia wards is, to be honest, not a place calling for bravery of the conventional sort. For the nursing staff perhaps it is. They need to be brave enough to exert discipline, to be able to say 'No', to make the mechanism work. For the family members and friends being brave is secondary; the foremost quality is patience: to endure, to be gentle and stoic. Love, St Paul reminds us, always protects, always trusts, always hopes, always perseveres. He'd got it right. He didn't say it was easy, either.

Every morning, as I came into the ward, Frome or Garden Court alike, I would kiss Ella and hold her hand. Once another lady, tall and good-looking, easily the youngest patient there, said to us, 'What is it like?'

Mystified I could only say, 'I'm sorry?' the familiar code-words for 'Could you explain that?'

'Being kissed. Is it nice?'

'Yes,' said Ella.

'No-one has ever kissed me,' she said.

She leaned back in her chair and that was that. She still looked in our direction, but it was the familiar unfocused look, simply her face by chance directed our way. I felt uneasily that something had been left unsaid, some small kindness not offered. But for mortals such as I one unreachable star was enough.

Though we ventured out almost every day there were also times when we did spend hours in the wards. The big concerts were always good value, though Garden Court had its own smaller occasions when the dozen or so patients gathered, for instance, to be entertained by a jolly man with an electronic keyboard. A lady pianist led our small group in singing, even providing songbooks which somehow gave the impression of having originally hailed from the United States, about the time of the Civil War. We sang *Dixie, My Grandfather's Clock, The Yellow Rose of Texas* among others. Ella, who had once been a fine singer, joined in quietly but often urged me to take a leading role, on the grounds of being the only male voice. As a mediocre singer, at best, I thought it wise to discourage this, but did once, against my better judgement, lead our shaky voices thus:

Come and sit by my side if you love me,
Do not hasten to bid me adieu,
But remember the Red River valley...

Ella who, as always, was sitting by my side, thoroughly approved of the words. She died not long after this occasion, though never realising the proximity of death. She was, in those final months, confident and at ease, her magic regenerated, her aura unchallenged.

My mind has retained much of those final months. Ella's room was functional with a large ensuite bathroom. After her third fall in June 2015 she could no longer go home, unable to climb the steep terrace steps to our door. So I filled her room with her tapestries, with photographs of her in all her young vigour and beauty, and always brought flowers and chocolates, of which she particularly approved.

In fact she accepted her room but far preferred that we go outside on our daily wheelchair treks. I discovered a subsidised Adelaide municipal service which provided large taxis into which she could be wheeled while still in her chair; then the driver would take us to various destinations and collect us later. As a destination Botanic Park always met with her approval and she was delighted to attend her younger grandson's confirmation at St Peter's College chapel.

To her room and the communal lounge alike she was indifferent. There was a sort of cycle of entertainment, so that one heard and saw on the screen various items, more or less daily. Omnipresent was *The Sound of Music*. There were other regulars such as *Singing in the Rain* and *The Wizard of Oz*. Ella paid little attention though did cast an interested eye on *River Dance*, an Irish dancing show, perhaps recalling how long ago she'd tacked on to a dancing line in Galway, as lissom and Hibernian as anyone.

One understood that soothing and familiar items made sense and only once was I mindless enough to say 'Please, no,' when 'High on a hill was a lonely goatherd' struck up.

'What would you prefer, John?' said a diminutive Indian nurse.

'Just a change. It doesn't have to be *Apocalypse Now.*'

'*Apocalypse Now* would not be appropriate, John.'

There was also a collection of songs that filled the gap between *The Sound of Music* and *The King and I,* eventually hypnotising me into singing along with 'Daddy wouldn't buy me a bow-wow! Bow-wow!'

Ella generally forbade this: 'Stick to the Red River Valley,' she said.

'Come and sit by my side if you love me...'

'That's better,' she said.

'Can I sing "A soldier was saying goodbye to his horse"?'

'I don't think I know that.' Of course. It was far too recent, we needed to be sixty years back, safe where the memories were intact, back where a nervous nineteen-year-old boy had asked her if she would like to go for a walk.

Our most frequent visits were to O'Connell Street, where we almost became an institution. In at least three restaurants someone would be there to hold the door open as we approached, or even take the chair from me and wheel it inside. Ella liked, almost to the very end, to go out for lunch and afternoon tea. One such occasion will never leave me, not least in that it told me that the gall and wormwood she had drunk over my ludicrous 'infidelity' were gone, exorcised, and the world was a better place. We went into the Palazzo at the north end of O'Connell Street. By this time my continual years-long presence seemed to have reassured her that her magnetism and feminine aura had not deserted her, as indeed they had not. Angela, who appeared to run the place, would spot us at the entrance and rush out to help me haul the wheelchair inside. Ella always chose lemon gelato. She liked to give me the small spoon and whisper: 'Help me with the ice cream,' though needing no help whatever. She would put her tongue out, waiting for me to put a dab of ice cream on it then slowly slide it into her mouth, all the time looking directly into my eyes and fluttering her eyelashes. It was an action so overtly flirtatious, so coquettish, it was mesmerising.

On other days we stopped at a particular coffee shop, notable for their iced tarts each decorated with a crystallised cherry. Again she would put out her tongue, encourage me to place a cherry on it, then balance it into her mouth. As a ritual it was tantalising and seductive. And there was I thinking the ball would never hit a red slot again. Five years and nothing but black.

'I love you,' I said.

'I know,' she said. Croupier, hand me the jackpot.

XXX

Gradually Ella grew weaker, until the wheelchair was replaced with a contraption which was essentially a bed on wheels. This provided a pillow for her to rest her head, while still allowing me to take her for walks. Though she was as keen as ever to go out of the ward the bed-cum-trolley was too heavy to go far and sadly our walks were restricted to about a quarter of a mile. We could not access anywhere even for a cup of tea other than Helping Hand's café. Spring had come and we liked to choose a route that passed under several jacaranda trees, then in full bloom. She liked the blue petals to drift down and stay on her blankets.

December the 7th, 2015 was a Monday. As usual I arrived about eleven o'clock. Unusually a nurse said, 'I'll go with you to her room.' My dearest girl was unconscious, breathing in long, laboured, sobbing gasps which shook her whole frame.

'How long has it been like this?' I said.

'Since about four hours ago.'

'Has the doctor been...?'

'Yes.'

'...and he says?'

'She is dying. I'm sorry.'

There seemed nothing left to say. The nurse left. A few moments later the matron came in.

'What are you going to do?' she asked.

'Stay here,' I said. 'We've got a lot to talk about.'

So I stayed until eight in the evening, for she did not leave our world easily. Nor did it surprise me, for she was a born fighter. Though moment by moment it seemed each racking, body-shaking breath would be her last, it was not so. Each time there was a pause so that literally thousands of times in the next nine hours I wondered where she would find the strength for one more breath, one more shuddering inhalation.

For safety reasons the bed was low and I found a small stool and crouched on it, bent over the bed. After several hours a painful cramp set in, so I knelt on the floor. This was better as now I could put my arms around her. Every hour or so a nurse brought in a cup of tea or coffee and once I went to the little café and bought a packet of biscuits.

Very early, on this the saddest of days, my thoughts had turned to how on my hospital visits, as an undergraduate, to my cousin Tom, after his fighter aircraft crashed, I had tried to speak to him, unconscious though he was, and a nurse had encouraged me.

'Somewhere deep down, he can hear you,' she said.

So I set out to talk to my love and it lasted nine hours. Of course I never finished, because it would have needed ninety or nine hundred hours or more to relate our love story.

'Do you remember ... do you remember...?' She would remember I knew and clearly, in itself a defiance of Alzheimer's. The disease had certainly eroded our marriage for a while but somehow the pernicious central delusion had dissipated.

In January 2018, two years and a month after Ella's death, my brother had told me of the fate of one of my best and closest friends. Jeff and I went to primary school together, camped out in the woods together when we were eight or nine, ran in and out of one another's houses, played together in junior and senior sporting teams where I always admired his skill and spirit. Like my brother he spent all his working life in one of Lincoln's steel foundries. He was a friend I was glad to have. He died of Alzheimer's, interned, knowing nothing and nobody, in some god-forsaken puzzled loneliness. Earlier I told you of my day-dream of the carefree little lads paddling in the bright stream, poised airily for their bright futures. One of them was Jeff.

Somehow my girl was spared this grim end and everything I reminded her of I believe she heard.

I know you'll never forget Walnut Place, your parents, brothers and sisters, South Park school and fighting on the first morning. 'Keep fighting,' I said. 'We've so much to recall. Don't leave me.' Just think back to fetching coal in a bathtub, the newspaper round, maths and Latin, the poetry of John

Milton that you quoted so easily, the prose of Jane Austen, your prizes, the evenings you went dancing, playing hockey for England with the red rose on your shirt.

Do you remember the moment you walked in, dazzling and disturbing, to the Tax Office's filing room, remember our first walks, first kiss, the photo you gave me. Yes, I've still got it. The pheasant I brought you.

And the encounter in Silver Street, you with your basket of potatoes and onions, and picking violets in my uncle's wood, then you the belle of the May Ball in your ice-blue dress, our snowed-in wedding, my hunting liquorice for you in the snow-storm, our baby coming. It's all right, I know you remember it all.

And Rhodesia, and Lucia and Nimrod and Ezekiel and the witchdoctor, Victoria Falls, the elephants, Madeleine being born, the Karoo and you jumping in the guard's van with the train moving.

Think back to Grasby, Guy Fawkes nights, Christmases, the bees, the little school, Snow White and the marrows, snow on the wolds, coal-fires, knowing we would never grow old.

Can you recall the people, the places, the wonderful multi-layered, many-coloured world we walked through together, not forgetting the shared worlds with our parents, our children and our grandchildren.

Then Australia's wide brown immensity with its shining coastal cities, a land that let you and your children reach high, for you a new profession and new perspectives.

The day wore on. Grief had so confounded my mind that by six o'clock words didn't seem to matter any more, or at least my words. So I ended my disjointed montage of memories and instead I knelt by the bedside with my arms around her and simply whispered her name. 'Ella' could be repeated two or three times between each rasping intake of breath.

She had, I knew

... come to the borders of sleep
The unfathomable deep
Forest where all must lose
Their way, however straight
Or winding, soon or late;

They cannot choose.

My thoughts were drawn to the blessed nights where she would speculate on what lay ahead for us. Generally she meant only our plans for the near future but there were also deeper thoughts. Those were the nights when I called her 'Red', usually restricted to when we spoke of the cross-roads where love and death intersect.

The senior nurse came in about eight o'clock that night. 'You should go home now,' she said. I gave her my son's phone number and went round to his house, it being nearer to the hospital than was our house in Skye.

The phone call came about twenty minutes later. Our son took it. 'Mum is dead,' he said. How clear it all is, yet another eidetic memory, the glass I was drinking from rattling against my teeth, as if I couldn't move it away. Another half hour or so and she would have died in my arms. Not alone.

How does T.S Eliot say the world ends? 'Not with a bang but a whimper.' Sorry, fine poet he may be, but he's got this wrong. It ends with an 'if only'. Any gambler will tell you that.

Her cabin'd ample spirit
It fluttered and failed for breath.
Tonight it doth inherit
The vasty hall of death.

'You should sleep here,' said Kristen, our daughter-in-law. 'Have Alex's room.' So I went upstairs at once, grateful to be alone.

It was unlikely that sleep would come soon, if at all, so I picked up a book from my grandson's bedside cupboard. It was Michael Hussey's cricketing autobiography. A chapter in and the universe tilted on its axis. Ella's voice spoke. It came from the open window, almost as if she were perched on the window-sill. There was only one word spoken. It was my name. Its tone was her affectionate banter, as if she might soon say, 'How could anyone fail maths?'

Never before had the transcendental touched me. My immediate reaction was to try to deal rationally with the phenomenon. For a start was I dreaming? Absolutely not. If anything it was the opposite, being awake and alert, certainly enough to grasp that this wanted every atom of my thought and concentration. For instance, where exactly had the voice come from? Somewhere near the open window. Then, as it was monosyllabic, what other sound might it have been? A dog? A bird-call? A car? No, clearly none of these. So perhaps a stress-induced hallucination. No, not even close. I was thinking icily clearly, and my mind felt a total certainty that I'd eliminated every possibility but one, so the one was the truth.

The truth is usually uncomplicated. It was what it was. Later I told Ella's close friend, June, who, to my surprise, took it in her stride. 'It happens,' she said. How privileged I was and am.

Thereafter only the conventional. Thanks to the generous co-operation of the headmaster, her funeral in the chapel of St Peter's College was all it should have been. My son, son-in-law, grandsons and I carried her coffin from the chapel. It seemed eerily distant, as if I were observing the ritual from afar. My heart was sick, longing for the ripple of her voice and the lost delight of her closeness.

Her ashes, as she instructed me, I took to England. 'Let me rest not far from my mother,' she had said, 'and next to you.' It was a perfect English morning, the sky blue and Washingborough churchyard quiet, green and secluded. It could easily have been June in any of the centuries since people first worshipped there. The service, which took place outside, was simple and moving. As we stood with our feet in the daisies my parents' graves were perhaps four paces away, and nearby were those of my grandparents, uncle and cousins. My dashing cousin Barbara's grave was still freshly dug, heaped with funeral wreaths. She had fought the Alzheimer demon to the very end.

Ah, God! that it were possible
For one short hour to see
The souls we loved, that they
might tell us
What and where they be...

The little service ended and suddenly the church bells pealed and echoed across the Lincolnshire countryside, the words of John Bunyan springing into truth:

So [s]he passed over and all the trumpets sounded for her on the other side.

A sandstone block marks her grave, with room next to it for me to join her. *Who said, 'Where sleeps she now Where rests she now her head Bathed in eve's loveliness.' That's what I said.*

The stone is inscribed:
Ella Roe

1934–2015

Beloved.

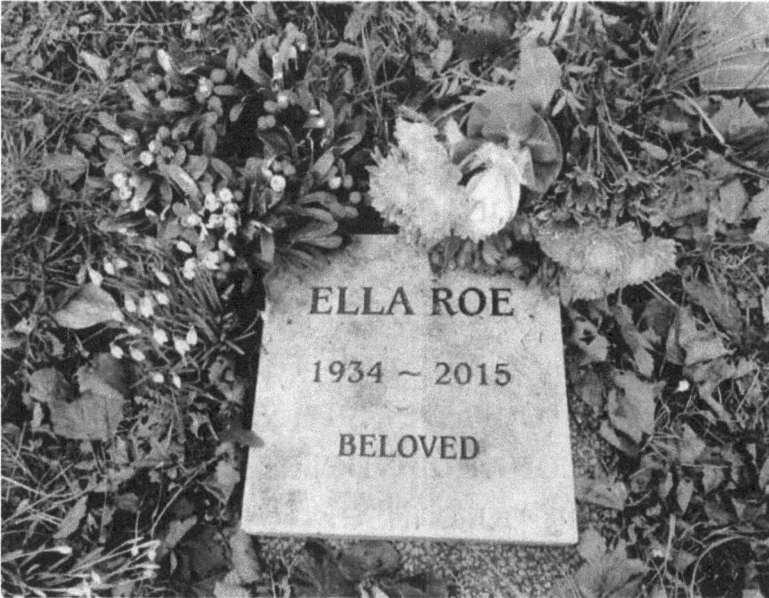

BACK COVER MATERIAL

John Roe's witty and lyrical memoir is an almost-perfect love story ... until the arrival of the demon.

As a bright young student, future English teacher John found Ella, a woman who both matched his intellect and would help keep his feet on the ground. Together, they shared a wonderful marriage: they were lucky.

But when Ella began to slip into dementia, their good fortune turned ferociously dark.

John labels the dementia that stole his wife as 'the demon': a malevolent force that destroys lives and extinguishes happiness. British neuroscientist Joseph Jebelli predicts that dementia will, unless we find a cure, affect one third of the world population over the next seven decades. Until there is a way to cure or prevent it, the 'demon' of dementia must be faced down.

This passionate, immersive memoir takes the reader inside an emotional rollercoaster of losing a loved one to an outside force you can neither halt nor control.

* 9 7 8 0 3 6 9 3 8 7 1 5 8 *